P9-CML-153

HOW TO MANAGE YOUR CHILD'S LIFE-THREATENING FOOD ALLERGIES

PRACTICAL TIPS FOR EVERYDAY LIFE

VALLEY COTTAGE
LIBRARY
Valley Cottage
New York 10989

Linda Marienhoff Coss

Plumtree Press acknowledges that similar information has also been previously published by The Food Allergy and Anaphylaxis Network (FAAN) in their various educational materials, and is grateful for FAAN's contributions to this book.

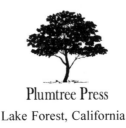

Plumtree Press
Lake Forest, California

HOW TO MANAGE YOUR CHILD'S
LIFE-THREATENING FOOD ALLERGIES

PRACTICAL TIPS FOR EVERYDAY LIFE

———⟋❦⟍———

Plumtree Press/May, 2004

All rights reserved.
Copyright © 2004 by Linda Marienhoff Coss.

Text Design by Robin Smith
Cover Design by Ken Harris

No part of this book may be reproduced or transmitted in any form
or by any means, electronic or mechanical, including photocopying,
recording or by any information storage or retrieval system, except as
may be expressly permitted by law or in writing from the publisher,
or except by a reviewer who may quote brief passages in review
to be printed in a magazine or newspaper.

Permission should be addressed in writing to:
Plumtree Press
P.O. Box 1313, Lake Forest, California 92609-1313
or to permissions@FoodAllergyBooks.com.

Although the author and publisher have strived to ensure the
accuracy and completeness of the information contained in this book,
we assume no responsibility for errors, inaccuracies, omissions or
any inconsistency herein.

Library of Congress Catalog Card Number: 2003098036

ISBN 0-9702785-1-9

Printed in the United States of America

DEDICATION

I dedicate this book to my parents,
Diana and Steve,
who "get it,"
and are always there for me;
and to my children....
Jason,
who tackles his unique challenges
with style and grace,
and Kevin,
whose passion and enthusiasm
fills our household.

ALSO BY LINDA COSS

What's to Eat?
The Milk-Free, Egg-Free, Nut-Free
Food Allergy Cookbook

ACKNOWLEDGEMENTS

Writing this book has been an enormous project, and I could not have done it without the support and input of many people.

I would like to offer a heartfelt thank you to The Food Allergy & Anaphylaxis Network (FAAN) for reviewing my manuscript, granting me reprint permission for a wide variety of materials, and encouraging me throughout this project. Much of the information presented in this book has also been published in various ways and formats by FAAN, and I can't thank FAAN enough for the wonderful work that they've done in the areas of food allergy education and advocacy.

Thank you also to Chris Papkee of PeanutAllergy.com for your comments and insights; and to the food allergy organizations around the world which so generously reviewed my manuscript and provided an "international perspective" – Anaphylaxis Australia, Allergy New Zealand, the Anaphylaxis Campaign in the United Kingdom, and the Allergy/Asthma Information Association in Canada.

I would like to thank all of my "food allergy friends" who shared their stories and their advice with me. This includes many of my support group friends – Anjali, Barbara, Diane, Erica, Gay and her daughter Ariella, Heidi and her daughter Marlee, Janet, Lauralyn, Leslie, Michelle, and Tanya; as well as many other moms across the country and around the globe that I was fortunate to speak or correspond with – Angela in Northern California, Ann in Wisconsin, Donna in Minnesota, Gail in Pennsylvania, Joann in Virginia, Julie in South Carolina, Laura in Northern California, Michelle in Minnesota, Raniah in South Carolina, Samantha in Southern California, Pamela in Spain, and Jackie in Australia.

I would like to thank my mother, Diana Marienhoff, and my friends, Catherine Balck, Barbara Elter and Lauralyn Markle, for their editing and proofreading assistance; and of course Robin Smith for her wonderful graphic design. I would also like to thank Doug Tamkin for completely redesigning my website (www.FoodAllergyBooks.com) in honor of this new book.

And last – but never least – I would like to thank my children, Jason and Kevin, for being patient while I devoted so much of my time and energy to this project.

LEGAL DISCLAIMER

The information contained in this book is not intended to replace the advice of your child's physician, nor is it meant to replace medical diagnosis or treatment. If you have or suspect that your child has food allergies, you are strongly urged to seek out appropriate medical advice. If your child is already under the care of a physician for food allergies, be sure to discuss with him or her any changes that you intend to make in the management of your child's food allergies.

Each child's condition is different, and the information presented in this book may or may not be appropriate for your child.

No promises or warranties, express or implied, as to the appropriateness of any information or advice for the management of a particular person's food allergies is made by this book. No liability will be assumed by anyone affiliated with the writing, production or distribution of this book for any damages arising from the information presented herein, whether such losses are special, incidental, consequential, or otherwise.

The reader accepts sole responsibility for the use of the information contained in this book.

TABLE OF CONTENTS

MY STORY

In many respects, my story is probably quite similar to yours. My initial reaction to my son's diagnosis was one of shock and disbelief. I struggled to cope with the necessary changes in my family's lifestyle before I eventually adjusted to what essentially is a different way of life. I have spoken to many parents of food-allergic children, and in so many ways we have all had rather similar experiences.

As an author, though, I feel compelled to share my particular story with you anyway. I want you to know me, to know the path that led me to writing this book. And I want an excuse to write something emotional, before I get into the very non-emotional, straight-forward advice of the rest of this book!

My story begins in 1991….

I sat nervously in the chair in front of the doctor's desk, trying desperately to calm my wailing toddler. Jason was only 18 months old, but he had already developed such a dread of doctors and doctors' offices and tests and shots that he became hysterical at the mere sight of a waiting room. He had vomited when we entered the examination room. And now he was crying uncontrollably.

"Mrs. Coss," I heard the doctor say, "This is one of the three worst sets of test results that I have seen in my twenty years of practice."

And so began my journey into the world of food allergies.

Through trial and error I had already discovered that Jason reacted to milk products, eggs and nuts. Even in my naïve "first-time mother" state, I knew that something was wrong when a child spontaneously broke out in hives during lunch. But I had no inkling of the depth of the now blood test-confirmed problem.

"Based on these test results," continued the doctor, "I believe Jason is at high risk for anaphylaxis."

"Anaphy-what?" I thought.

"If Jason were to consume an allergen," he explained, "even a tiny amount of allergen, he could go into anaphylactic shock. This is a very serious condition which can rapidly lead to death – within minutes or hours."

"WHAT???" I thought, holding Jason just a little closer, "did he say DEATH???"

I don't clearly remember the rest of the conversation. I don't think I truly heard it.

By the time the appointment ended I had learned that there was no cure for food allergies and that the only "treatment" was a "strict avoidance diet." I left the office armed with a syringe full of epinephrine and instructions on how to use it if Jason had an allergic reaction, a long list of ingredients to avoid (who would have thought that "milk" could be called so many different things?), a collection of informational pamphlets, contact information for a dietician, a whimpering toddler (exhaustion was finally setting in), and an unshakable urge to scream and cry hysterically.

It didn't take long – perhaps a few weeks – for me to fully understand Jason's diagnosis, and to understand that screaming and crying hysterically probably was an appropriate response.

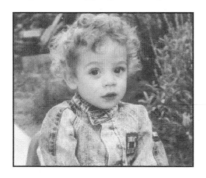

From the food allergy perspective, Jason was an ultra-sensitive child. I quickly discovered that Jason was so exquisitely sensitive that he would develop hives around his mouth within 30 seconds of consuming a tiny bite of a food that was merely produced on the same machinery as another product that contained a tiny amount of an allergen!

This was ridiculous. All I could think was that if exposure to a practically microscopic quantity of allergen produced an immediate (although minor) reaction, what would happen if he actually had a mouthful of milk or a bite of peanut butter? Anaphylaxis – and possible death – was a very real possibility.

This was when the depth of the problem truly began to set in. What did it mean to parent a toddler who was at risk for literally dropping dead if he consumed a tiny amount of the wrong food? It meant reading the ingredient panel of every single food item that I purchased, every time I purchased it. For me it also meant cooking everything from scratch and avoiding restaurants, because back then I wasn't able to obtain reliable ingredient or cross-contamination information from either food manufacturers or restaurant managers.

The more time went on, the more issues I discovered. Parenting this toddler meant never – and I mean never – allowing him to be more than an arm's distance away from me when we were not at home. As a toddler, he naturally had an innate need to grab everything in sight and shove it into his mouth. Social situations were a minefield. We encountered small children covered with cake and ice cream, dishes of nuts and colorful candies, tables full of forbidden food, relatives with food residue on their hands or lips wanting to touch or kiss Jason, and well-meaning people wanting to give the adorable little boy with the big brown eyes a bite of something delicious ("just one bite – a little bite can't possibly hurt anything").

Eventually, of course, I adjusted. I became adept at reading labels, I was a seasoned pro at picnic packing, I successfully convinced everyone in Jason's life that I wasn't exaggerating about the whole thing (Deadly food allergies? Preposterous! Who ever heard of such an absurdity?), I saved a lot of money by not eating out, and life went on – although in a somewhat paranoid, always on-alert kind of a way.

When Jason was 2-1/2 my second son was born. Knowing that this was in our gene pool, I took every possible precaution to try to prevent Kevin from developing food allergies. All of my efforts paid off – eventually. By the age of five, Kevin could eat anything. However, when he was around one he had a reaction and developed a measurable allergy (he went 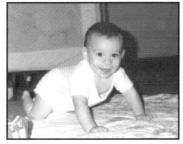 from "0" to the top-of-the-scale "4" on a "skin prick test") after consuming just a half a cup of milk and one egg! So it was back to my familiar mode of parenting: Staying within an arms' reach, carrying extra emergency medication, educating everyone in Kevin's life that he had this condition, too.

When Jason was 4 years old I started a local food allergy support group that has been a saving grace in my life ever since. Over the years our little group has hashed out solutions to most of the issues addressed in this book.

By the time the boys were a little older I became fed up with the lack of decent food allergy cookbooks that were then on the market. I decided to develop recipes and write my own. In December 2000 I published "What's to Eat? The Milk-Free, Egg-Free, Nut-Free Food Allergy Cookbook." I am extremely proud of the success of this book, and I am absolutely thrilled that my work has brought delicious food into the lives of thousands of families who thought their children were going to be limited to unappealing "special diet" fare.

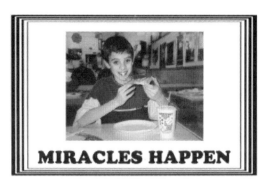

MIRACLES HAPPEN

In January 2002, at the age of 11-1/2, Jason outgrew his dairy allergy. To celebrate I threw the "Dairy Fest" party that I had been fantasizing about for years. We feasted on pizza, ice cream, cheese and crackers, and dairy-filled "party foods" of all kinds. The party invitation featured a picture of Jason with a piece of pizza dangling out of his smiling face. The caption read, "Miracles Happen."

In December 2002 I had a very long telephone conversation with a woman in Northern California who had called to ask advice about starting a support group in her area. Our conversation flowed from one food allergy-related topic to another, and she asked for input regarding how to handle a wide range of issues. It was actually her off-hand comment at the end of our conversation that I "ought to write a book with all this advice" that was the trigger for this entire project!

For many years now, one of my personal goals has been to make a positive difference in the lives of others and to do my part to help "heal the world." In this book I have provided practical advice on how to handle the wide variety of situations that face parents of food-allergic children. I sincerely hope that this advice helps you to keep your precious child safe and healthy, and that it makes your life in the food allergy world a little easier.

INTRODUCTION

Each year thousands of children around the world are diagnosed with life-threatening food allergies. Although it is nice to know that you're not alone, this fact really is of little comfort when the child in question is your child. **Your** child is not a statistic. And all of those thousands of other parents out there are not with you to help you deal with this very serious condition – but I am.

It is very, very frightening to be told that your child can die if he or she eats the wrong thing. It is even more frightening if your child is one of those for whom just touching – or even inhaling – an allergen can cause a reaction. If your child was recently diagnosed, you may not yet know just how sensitive he or she is. Regardless of the degree of sensitivity, however, a diagnosis of "anaphylactic" or life-threatening food allergies must be taken very seriously.

I have written this book to help **you** manage **your** child's life-threatening food allergies. I am not a doctor or a health professional. I am a fellow parent who has been living life in the "food allergy lane" for twelve years…managing my own child's allergies, running a local support group, and even writing and self-publishing a food allergy cookbook. Think of me as your neighbor and friend, your "personal support group leader" who will pave the way for you.

Food, of course, is everywhere. There is food in our homes, food in our friends' homes, and food at the shopping center. There's food at social gatherings, food at schools, food at playgrounds. Everywhere they go, people eat. And everywhere there is food, there is a potentially dangerous situation for your child.

As the parent of a child with life-threatening food allergies, you need to learn a new way to approach common, everyday situations. How do you determine which food is "safe" for your child and which is not? How do you handle social situations, school, and travel? Are there any potential dangers lurking at the playground, the movie theater, or your child's best friend's living room? And if there are potential dangers, what can you do to make the situation reasonably safe for your child?

As much as possible in this book, I have attempted to steer clear of "medical" advice. Explanations of allergy physiology, allergy testing and the latest medical research are all relatively easy to find on websites and in other books. My focus instead is on presenting practical tips and advice...the nitty-gritty details of how to live as full and "normal" a life as possible while keeping your child safe in a food-filled world.

You may not be aware that even among those whose allergies are so severe as to be labeled "potentially fatal," there is a wide degree of variation in food sensitivity. I know one peanut-allergic teenager, for instance, who can touch a food product to his tongue and "sense" whether or not the food is safe for him to eat – and he suffers no ill effects from touching the food in this way. Many, many other peanut-allergic individuals would be likely to have an anaphylactic reaction if their tongue touched a peanut-containing food. Some of the food-allergic have a reaction if an allergen merely touches their skin; others only react to what they eat. And there are those who suffer ill effects if they merely inhale the airborne particles of the offending food. Whether or not all of the advice in this book pertains to **your** child depends almost entirely on just how sensitive he or she is.

Based on your doctor's advice and your experience with your child, you will need to determine which precautions you need to take and which you can safely ignore. There are some precautions you will need to take when your child is very young that will not be necessary when he grows older. If your child is not exquisitely sensitive, some of the advice which I present in this book may seem rather extreme. Rest assured, however, that all of these precautions grew out of real-life situations which caused problems for food-allergic children.

The good news is that many children outgrow their food allergies, and for many others the situation at least improves over time. Today, for instance, your child may react if an allergen merely touches his skin. When he is older, it is possible that his skin sensitivity may decrease and he may only react to what he eats.

As of this writing, there is no "cure" for anaphylactic food allergies. Although researchers are working on a variety of very promising treatments, there is currently nothing that will make your child's condition miraculously disappear. The only "treatment" is complete avoidance of the allergen(s). And "completely avoiding" common food items can be easier said than done.

As your "personal support group leader" I want to warn you (and apologize in advance) that you are likely to feel completely overwhelmed – and possibly frightened – by the information presented in this book. This book is extremely detailed, and the sheer volume of information itself can be hard to take. You may be shocked to realize all of the precautions that you may need to take to keep your child safe. Plus, many of the tips I give are illustrated with fairly upsetting true stories from the lives of other food allergy families. I want to assure you, however, that all of this really will become second nature to you. It does get much easier over time.

Your child is precious, and – just like those thousands of other parents out there – you can successfully manage his or her life-threatening food allergies. Your child can eat and play and have fun, go to school, have friends. Your child can go to the movies, join the baseball team, and take music lessons. Your family can enjoy outings, vacations, and a social life. It all just takes a different approach, and a lot more advance planning, than it does for other families.

CHAPTER 1
PREPARING FOR AND TREATING SEVERE ALLERGIC REACTIONS

Your child has been diagnosed with "life-threatening food allergies." So what in the world does this mean? It means that your child is at risk for a potentially fatal systemic reaction called "anaphylaxis." This chapter will explain how to recognize and treat an anaphylactic reaction, and will discuss the basic steps that you need to take to be prepared to do so.

SYMPTOMS OF ANAPHYLAXIS

A food allergy is caused when a person's immune system mistakenly believes that a normally harmless substance – food – is harmful. When the individual eats the food (or, in some cases, merely touches the food or inhales particles of the food), the immune system releases massive amounts of chemicals and histamines. This in turn triggers a variety of allergic symptoms that can affect one or more of the body's systems, including the skin, respiratory system, gastrointestinal system, or cardiovascular system.

An anaphylactic reaction is a severe allergic reaction that, if not properly treated, can rapidly lead to death. Symptoms usually begin to appear within seconds to two hours after exposure to the allergen, and can include any or all of the following[1]:

✦ **MOUTH:** Itching, swelling, burning, and/or tingling of the lips, tongue, or mouth

✦ **THROAT:** Itching and/or a sense of tightness in the throat; hoarseness; hacking cough

✦ **SKIN:** Hives, itchy, and/or swelling about the face or extremities

✦ **GUT:** Nausea, abdominal cramps, vomiting, and/or diarrhea; loss of bowel control

✦ **LUNGS:** Shortness of breath, repetitive coughing, and/or wheezing

---

[1] Reprinted with permission from The Food Allergy and Anaphylaxis Network's "Food Allergy Action Plan" (See Appendix B).

✦ **HEART:**   "Thready" pulse; rapid and severe drop in blood pressure; loss of consciousness

✦ **OTHER:**   A frightening feeling that can be described as an "impending sense of doom"

It is important to keep in mind that during an anaphylactic reaction, your child's symptoms can rapidly progress from "bad to worse to horrible" literally within moments. One moment your child may be breaking out in hives, and in the time it takes you to say "oh my gosh, what's wrong with Susie?" and start to grab for her emergency medicine, she may progress to breathing difficulty and vomiting. Although reactions are not always this rapid and dramatic, they frequently are. Therefore, you must **always** be prepared for an emergency!

RECOGNIZING ANAPHYLAXIS

Most parents who have seen their child experience an anaphylactic reaction say that when "the big one" hits, you couldn't miss it. Their children were clearly in extreme distress. Occasionally, however, the symptoms start out more subtly and are more difficult to recognize.

When your child feels ill, vomits, continuously tries to clear her throat, or experiences a bout of asthma, you need to remember to assess whether or not the episode is being caused by an allergic reaction to food. Not all allergic reactions will involve hives or visible swelling.

> *When Michelle's daughter Ally was about 5 years old she took one bite of a piece of bread at a restaurant which had a sesame seed stuck to it and immediately started clearing her throat. Michelle gave her a sip of water. Ally continued the throat clearing. A few minutes later when Ally complained that she didn't feel well, Michelle saw that the whites of Ally's eyes were red, noticed that the pitch of her voice had changed, and realized that Ally was having an allergic reaction. Although she had no hives at all, Ally's throat was closing up.*

> *During a bout with a bad cold Laura's food-allergic toddler woke up from his nap with a cough. Owen took one sip of rice milk and immediately spit it up and coughed more. Laura figured he just couldn't drink anything until he'd woken up a bit. Then Owen coughed again and began throwing up. Then he repeatedly asked for his "puffer" (asthma inhaler), which he*

does not like. Laura figured her son was getting the flu. When Owen broke out in hives Laura finally "got it" that he was having an anaphylactic reaction. To what? The liquid in the sippy cup turned out to be cow's milk, not rice milk. His caregiver had made a mistake when she fixed the drink earlier in the day.

————— ❧ —————

Any time your child experiences **any** of the symptoms listed on page 11 you need to quickly assess the situation and immediately take the appropriate course of action. Stay with your child and monitor his condition until the reaction is completely over and he no longer shows any symptoms of an allergic reaction. If your child has asthma, remember that an allergic reaction can trigger his asthma, too either in addition to or instead of other symptoms. Speak with your child's physician regarding instructions on how and when to treat an asthma attack.

TREATING ANAPHYLAXIS

The "drug of choice" for initial treatment of a life-threatening anaphylactic reaction is injectable epinephrine, and (as of this writing) the preferred delivery system for this injection of epinephrine is an EpiPen®. An EpiPen® is a disposable, pre-filled automatic injection device which contains a single dose of epinephrine. It is easy to use and easy to carry, and is relatively non-threatening due to its lack of an exposed needle (the needle automatically ejects when the unit is activated). The EpiPen® can even be used through clothing, and the injection of epinephrine should improve your child's symptoms almost immediately. EpiPens® are only available by prescription.

————— ❧ —————

Note: Antihistamine by itself (either by prescription or over-the-counter) is not a treatment for anaphylaxis, but is usually given after the epinephrine injection.

————— ❧ —————

EpiPens® come in two strengths. The EpiPen® Jr. is for younger children. It contains one dose of 0.15 mg epinephrine, and has a shorter needle than the "regular" EpiPen®. The "regular" EpiPen® contains 0.30 mg epinephrine. Your child's doctor will decide which EpiPen® to prescribe based on your child's weight. As your child gets older and larger, be sure to talk to the physician regarding when to make the change from the EpiPen® Jr. to the EpiPen®.

Note: Throughout this book, I will refer to both the EpiPen® Jr. and the EpiPen® generically as the "EpiPen®." All instructions are identical for both.

———————

If your child is having an allergic reaction, you must act very quickly... preferably within seconds of when you realize there is something wrong. The sooner you act, the better the likelihood that the incident will have a positive resolution.

———————

Any time you use the EpiPen® you must immediately call the rescue squad and have your child transported to the hospital for further treatment and observation. The EpiPen® merely "buys" you time to get to the hospital. The effects of the EpiPen® might wear off in 10 to 20 minutes.

———————

Throughout this book, I refer to calling the "rescue squad" rather than an "ambulance." In the U.S., not all emergency workers are authorized to administer epinephrine. In those states that only grant this authorization to certain categories of emergency workers, ambulance drivers may not be able to assist you whereas paramedics (i.e., the workers in the "rescue squad") may.

———————

Always use the EpiPen® first and then call the rescue squad after you have given your child the injection. If your child is having an anaphylactic reaction, the EpiPen® must be used immediately, without any delay.

 INTERNATIONAL PERSPECTIVE

COUNTRY	COMMENTS
United Kingdom	In the U.K., you should call an ambulance rather than the "rescue squad." **Note:** Wherever the term "rescue squad" appears in this book, those in the U.K. should substitute "ambulance."

If the EpiPen® wears off and the symptoms return before you can get your child to the hospital, you can give a second injection 10 to 20 minutes after the first.

———✌———

Anaphylactic reactions can be "biphasic," which means that after the initial reaction is under control there is a good chance that the symptoms will reoccur 1 to 4 hours later. Therefore, after an anaphylactic reaction you need to stay at the hospital emergency room for at least 4 hours. If the hospital staff is not knowledgeable about this aspect of anaphylaxis and insists on discharging your child, you should stay on the hospital premises (such as in the waiting room) during this time period.

HOW TO USE AN EPIPEN®

It is best to lie your child down on his back for this procedure. If he is hysterical it will be easier to hold him down in this position; if he passes out before or during the injection he will not fall.

———✌———

If you are dealing with an uncooperative child, and another adult is available, have one person hold the child down while the other uses the EpiPen®.

———✌———

If you are dealing with an uncooperative child and you are on your own, you can gently lay your body across his (with your head facing his legs) hold one of his legs down with one hand, and inject the EpiPen® into the thigh of his other leg using your other hand. You may want to practice this maneuver (now – not during an emergency!) using a large stuffed animal.

———✌———

Although it is preferable to use the EpiPen® on bare skin, it can be used through clothing.

———✌———

Never put your thumb, fingers, or hand over the black tip of the EpiPen® unit.

DIRECTIONS FOR EPIPEN®USE² :

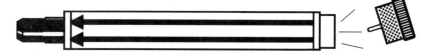

1. Do not remove the gray activation cap until ready to use.
2. Grasp EpiPen®, with the black tip pointing downward.
3. Form a fist around the EpiPen®, still keeping the black tip pointing downward.
4. With your other hand, pull off the gray activation cap.

Using EpiPen® Step 1   Using EpiPen® Step 2

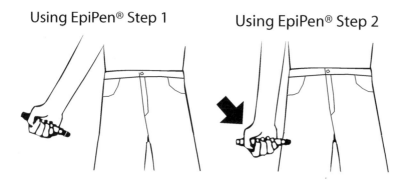

5. Hold black tip near child's outer thigh.
6. Swing and **jab firmly** into outer thigh so that the EpiPen® is perpendicular (at a 90 degree angle) to the thigh.
7. Hold **firmly in thigh** for 10 seconds (count "one one-thousand, two one-thousand" etc.)
8. Remove EpiPen® from thigh. Massage injection area for several seconds.
9. Check black tip of EpiPen®:
   a. If the needle is exposed, the dose was received.
   b. If not, repeat steps #5 – 8.
10. **Note:** Most of the liquid (about 90%) stays in the EpiPen® and cannot be reused.
11. Using a hard surface, bend the needle back against the EpiPen® unit.

² Reprinted with permission from Dey Corporation, from the EpiPen® Patient Insert.

12. Carefully put the EpiPen® (needle first) back into the carrying tube (without the gray activation cap).

13. Recap the carrying tube.

14. If prescribed by your child's physician, give your child a dose of antihistamine.

15. Call the rescue squad to immediately transport your child to the nearest hospital emergency room.

16. Tell the physician that you have administered an injection of epinephrine.

17. Give your used EpiPen® to the physician for inspection and proper disposal.

Although the EpiPen® needle looks as though it would be quite painful to use, I have spoken to children who say that the pain is actually quite minimal.

> *Ariella, age 11, had two anaphylactic episodes before it was determined that she had developed a new allergy. During the second reaction, she insisted on being the one to give the injection (although her mother was standing by). Ariella reports: "It doesn't really hurt very much, especially when I did it by myself. It made me feel much better about the way things were looking for my future when I will have to do it myself."*

AFTER AN ANAPHYLACTIC REACTION

If your child does have a serious reaction, learn from the experience. After your child is okay and you both have recuperated, review what went wrong. Try to figure out exactly what your child reacted to. If necessary, fine-tune your emergency action plan. And try not to berate yourself for the fact that the incident took place. Caring for a child with life-threatening food allergies can be an all-consuming task, and mistakes do happen.

> *Barbara points out that, for older children, having an "EpiPen® experience" helps reinforce that bad things do happen if you eat the wrong food. This becomes real rather than theoretical. In fact, her son Jake still talks about the reaction (and hospital Emergency Room visit) that he experienced five years ago.*

Remember, EpiPens® can only be used once. After you have used an EpiPen® you need to obtain a replacement.

CARING FOR EPIPENS®

EpiPens® should be stored in a dark place at room temperature (59-86 degrees Fahrenheit or 15 - 30 degrees Celsius). EpiPens® should not be refrigerated or exposed to extreme heat or cold.

———

If you order your EpiPens® from a mail-order pharmacy, be sure to inform the pharmacy that a signature must be required upon delivery. Otherwise, depending on the weather in your area on the day of delivery, the EpiPens® could be exposed to either freezing or very hot conditions as the package sits on your front porch, possibly causing the medication to be ruined.

———

EpiPens® are not good indefinitely. Each unit has an expiration date printed on it.

———

You should periodically examine the contents in the clear window of each of your child's EpiPen® units. If the solution is discolored or contains solid particles, you must replace the unit. Note that in an emergency, many physicians recommend use of an expired EpiPen® or an EpiPen® which has discolored contents rather than not administering any epinephrine at all. Speak to your child's physician before an emergency occurs regarding instructions for these situations.

———

In the United States, each EpiPen® comes with a registration form. Each time you purchase a new EpiPen® you should fill this form out and return it to the distributor. If you do so, you will receive an expiration reminder notice approximately one month before the EpiPen®'s expiration date. This is a free service, and a great "insurance policy" to make sure you replace your child's medication in a timely manner.

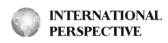

**INTERNATIONAL
PERSPECTIVE**

COUNTRY	COMMENTS
Australia	As of this writing, there is no EpiPen® registration service available in Australia, although it may become available.
Canada	The EpiPen® registration service is not available in Canada.
New Zealand	The EpiPen® registration service is not available in New Zealand.
United Kingdom	An EpiPen® registration service is available in the U.K.

EXPIRED EPIPENS®

Do not throw away your expired EpiPens®. Save these for use in practice sessions – just be sure to practice on an orange or grapefruit instead of on a person! Immediately after this "live ammunition" practice session you should safely dispose of both the fruit (I recommend cutting it up and running it through your garbage disposal) and the used EpiPen®.

CALLING THE RESCUE SQUAD

If your child is having an anaphylactic reaction, unless you live in a remote area where emergency response time is very slow, it is usually best to call the rescue squad or an ambulance rather than driving him to the hospital yourself. You are not likely be able to focus on driving safely while worrying about whether or not your child will live until you get him to the hospital.

Remember, **first** administer the EpiPen® and **then** call for help.

WHAT NUMBER TO DIAL

Emergency response systems differ from country to country. In the U.S., always dial 911.

 INTERNATIONAL PERSPECTIVE

COUNTRY	DIAL	COMMENTS
Australia	000	Specify that someone is having an anaphylactic reaction so that an intensive care ambulance, which is equipped with epinephrine, will be dispatched.
Canada	0 or the local ambulance number	Most ambulances in Canada carry epinephrine and at least one person who can inject it.
New Zealand	111	State "Ambulance" to be connected to the ambulance service. Specify that someone is having an anaphylactic reaction and that adrenaline is needed.
United Kingdom	999	For emergency services (ambulance, police, fire brigade), dial 999. In this case, specify that someone is having an anaphylactic reaction and needs adrenaline.

LEARN ABOUT YOUR LOCAL EMERGENCY RESPONSE SYSTEM

Long before an actual emergency happens, you should call whatever government agency is in charge of your local emergency medical response system (this may be the fire department, police department, or some other agency) to find out how emergency calls are handled in your area.

For example, in my city calls to 911 first go to the police dispatcher. We have been told that if we need to call 911 the first thing we should say is: "This is a medical emergency." The police dispatcher will immediately transfer the call to the fire dispatcher, who is responsible for dispatching the paramedics.

While you have this agency on the line, you should also find out what their policies are regarding administering medication to a child who is in anaphylactic shock. According to FAAN, as of this writing, for example, not all emergency response technicians in the United States are authorized to carry or use epinephrine. Some cannot use it at all, and others do not carry it but can help you administer **your** EpiPen® (which you should have used before calling the rescue squad in the first place).

I spoke to a woman who said that in her area the paramedics carry and are authorized to use epinephrine, but the Emergency Medical Technicians do not. She was told that when calling for help she must clearly state that her child is in anaphylactic shock and requires the paramedics and an ambulance. Otherwise, the less-prepared EMT's will be sent.

You may want to call your local paramedics to make sure that they are specifically aware of your child and are knowledgeable about anaphylaxis. Some areas even have a "registry" system whereby you can register your child with the local emergency medical authorities (although this may not be the case where you live).

CALLING FOR HELP

Keep an "emergency script" by each of your phones for use in case your child has an anaphylactic reaction at home. You (or the babysitter, or your child's sibling, or whoever) may find it difficult during the emergency to keep a clear head and think of what to say when calling for the rescue squad. See Appendix K for a sample script.

After calling for help, if you are not alone with your child, ask another adult or an older child to wait outside the building to flag down the rescue squad and direct them to your child. When they arrive, tell them that your child has severe food allergies, is experiencing an anaphylactic reaction, and that you have administered an EpiPen®.

CALLING FOR HELP USING A MOBILE TELEPHONE

In addition to always carrying your child's emergency medication pack (see pages 22-27) with you whenever you and your child leave the house, it is a good idea to also carry a cellular or mobile phone which you could use to call for help in an emergency.

———— ✊ ————

Long before an actual emergency happens, find out how emergency calls made from mobile phones are handled in your area, as these calls may be handled differently than calls from stationary phones.

> *Angela lives in a rural area in Northern California. She has been told that calls to 911 from her cellular phone will be answered by the Highway Patrol, and that there may be a significant delay before the call is answered and then transferred to the appropriate agency. In an emergency, she will receive a faster response if she calls an ambulance company directly. Angela therefore carries the telephone numbers of the local ambulance companies.*

MEDICINE PACK

If your child has potentially anaphylactic allergies it is imperative that her emergency medication is **always readily available**, whether she is at home or away from home. To make this happen you need to create a convenient and clearly labeled "medicine pack" to keep in a designated location at home and to bring with you whenever your child leaves the house.

———— ✊ ————

Of course, it is not enough to simply have the emergency medication available. There must also always be someone on hand who is knowledgeable about how and when to use it!

CONTENTS OF MEDICINE PACK

If your child has potentially anaphylactic allergies for which her doctor has prescribed an EpiPen®, you should have two EpiPens® readily available at all times. There are two reasons for this. First, it is statistically possible that an EpiPen® may malfunction. Second, an EpiPen® "buys" you 10 to 20 minutes to get your child to the hospital. You may need to use the second one before you get to the hospital or before the rescue squad arrives. If you carry EpiPens® with different lot numbers you also guard against the (statistically unlikely) possibility of something being wrong with a particular lot.

I recommend that your child's medicine pack contain the following:

2 EpiPens®, with different lot numbers

Whichever liquid antihistamine your child's doctor has prescribed (do not carry tablets — the liquid form is more rapid-acting)

A non-breakable plastic medicine server for serving the liquid antihistamine, clearly marked with the correct dosage. The little measuring cups that come with over-the-counter liquid antihistamines do not hold up well, and are likely to become cracked or broken. Appropriate medicine servers can be purchased at your local pharmacy.

Written instructions for how to recognize and treat an allergic reaction (see Appendix B)

A copy of your child's medical insurance card

Emergency contact numbers for you, your spouse, your child's doctors, etc.

A signed "Authorization to Consent to Treatment of a Minor" Form (See Appendix F), with the name of the adult being authorized to consent to the treatment left blank

Optional: You may also wish to include a few individually wrapped wet wipes in the medicine pack. This way you will always have something available with which to "wash" your child's hands before he eats or any time he touches something suspicious.

If your child has asthma, you should carry the asthma medication as well. If your child uses a nebulizer, you can carry a portable battery-operated model (although due to its size this will need to be carried outside of the medicine pack)

Place all of the paperwork that is in the medicine pack in a sealed zipper-type plastic bag to protect it from spills.

———— ❧ ————

If your child uses a spacer with the asthma inhaler, consider keeping the inhaler uncapped, inserted into the spacer, and ready to use.

While Laura's son Austin was playing at a friend's house he had an allergic reaction that triggered his asthma. The friend's mother gave Austin his inhaler, and then immediately called Laura. When Laura arrived she found that Austin's asthma had not improved. This was no surprise, as the other mother had not uncapped the inhaler prior to inserting it into the spacer!

Open fresh bottles of liquid over-the-counter antihistamines as soon as you get them home from the store, before you put them in a medicine pack or medicine cabinet. In the stress of an emergency it can be quite difficult to remove all of the safety packaging.

ALWAYS CARRY THE MEDICINE PACK

No matter where your child goes, his or her emergency medication must be available. Don't ever leave home without the medicine pack! Emergencies are never planned.

———————

You may wish to purchase a fanny pack (for you to wear) in which to carry your child's medicine pack.

> *Heidi has two medicine kits which she takes with her when her family leaves the house. The first is a large, insulated heat-proof/cold-proof container in which she keeps "everything," including a portable nebulizer. This kit stays in the car (when they're away from home or the hotel) or the hotel room (when they are at the hotel). The second is a fanny pack in which she carries the basic "medicine pack" items which I have listed above.*

 INTERNATIONAL PERSPECTIVE

COUNTRY	COMMENTS
Australia, New Zealand and United Kingdom	In Australia, New Zealand and the U.K., "fanny packs" are called "bum bags." Therefore, wherever the term "fanny pack" appears in this book, those in Australia, New Zealand or the U.K. should substitute the phrase, "bum bag."

To help you remember to always take the medicine pack with you when you leave the house, keep it somewhere that you're likely to see it when you're getting ready to leave, such as next to your car keys, purse or wallet. However, always keep it out of reach of babies and young children.

———————

Work out a system with your spouse to ensure that each of you always remembers to take the medicine pack on outings, and that each of you remembers to place the medicine pack back in its official "parking place" when you return home.

———— ❧ ————

Remember, EpiPens® should be kept at room temperature. Do not store your child's medicine pack in the car (which can get too hot or too cold, depending on the season and where you live) or in the refrigerator. It is okay to have the medicine in the car while you drive from place to place, but you should take it out of the car when you arrive at your destination.

———— ❧ ————

Of course, you should not leave your child's medicine pack in the car once you arrive at your destination anyway, because then it would not be with you!

CARRYING THE MEDICINE PACK
IN SUB-FREEZING WEATHER

If you are going to be out in the snow in sub-freezing temperature, you need to take extra care to ensure that the EpiPens® do not freeze. Avoid being out for long lengths of time. Wear the EpiPens® in a fanny pack close to your body, underneath your warm jacket. When you go back indoors, check each EpiPen® to ensure that the medication has not become cloudy or dis-colored.

CHECK THE EXPIRATION DATES

Be sure to periodically check the contents and expirations dates of all of your medicine packs. You should do this at least once every six months. Try to remember to check the medicine packs every time the clocks change, or at the start of Winter Break and Summer Vacation. While you're at it, this is a good time to also change the batteries in your home smoke detectors!

PREPARE EXTRA MEDICINE PACKS

If necessary, create an extra pack so that you and your spouse will each have one. If, for example, you usually drop your child off at school or day care in the morning and your spouse is responsible for the end-of-day pick up, you should each have a medicine pack. Do not rely on leaving the one medicine pack at school in the morning for your spouse to remember to pick up in the afternoon. What if he or she forgets?

Prepare an additional medicine pack to be kept with your earthquake, storm, or other emergency supplies (as appropriate for the region in which you live).

―――――― ⚓ ――――

Your child's school and/or day care provider should have medicine pack(s) which are kept on the premises. Have one pack that you carry with you, and at least one other that is always kept at school.

MEDICINE PACKS FOR OLDER CHILDREN

When your child gets older, you will need to start transitioning her to being responsible for carrying her own EpiPens®. The transition to the Middle School/Junior High School years (ages 11 to 14) is often an appropriate time to make this change.

 **INTERNATIONAL
PERSPECTIVE**

COUNTRY	COMMENTS
United Kingdom	At age 11, children go from Middle School to Secondary School. As of this writing, most Secondary Schools in the U.K. prefer youngsters to carry at least one EpiPen® with them.

To make it easier for your child to carry her medication, you can have her wear it in a fanny pack. By having the medication in something that is always kept on her person (as compared to in a purse or backpack), you eliminate a number of potential problems: the medication will not be set down somewhere, forgotten and then left behind; the medication will not be accessible to other children; and in an emergency the medication will always be very close at hand.

―――――― ⚓ ――――

There are a variety of specialty products designed for this purpose that are available through the Food Allergy and Anaphylaxis Network (FAAN) and various websites. You can purchase special fanny packs, belt packs, EpiPen® holders that clip onto a belt loop, non-breakable EpiPen® holders (that you would then insert into the fanny pack), and more.

My son began wearing his fanny pack to school and to away-from-home outings when he was in sixth grade. I opted for a regular fanny pack rather than a special EpiPen® holder because I did not feel that the available special carriers were large enough. Jason's fanny pack contains two EpiPens®, liquid Benadryl®, a medicine dispenser for taking the Benadryl®, written instructions for treating an allergic reaction, a copy of his medical insurance card, and home, work and cell phone numbers for both me and his father. All of the papers are in a sealed plastic bag to protect them from spills and leaks. When Jason becomes more socially independent I also intend to purchase a cellular phone for him to carry in his fanny pack as well.

Unless your school district already has an accommodating policy in place, you are likely to face an uphill battle when you announce that you want your child to carry (i.e., wear) his emergency medication. Even in states which have legislation in place specifically allowing children to carry life-saving medication, you may need to fight for your child's rights.

Our school district has strict "zero tolerance" policies – with very serious associated disciplinary actions – regarding children having any type of medicine, weapon, or potential weapon in their possession. An EpiPen® contains medication and a potential weapon (the needle). Luckily our district also has an official protocol in place for students to obtain permission to carry EpiPens®. In order to obtain this permission Jason's allergist and I had to provide recent allergy test results and fill out a seemingly endless pile of paperwork. In addition, Jason has been instructed not to tell other students what is in his fanny pack and not to show his EpiPens® to other students. The school is concerned that other students may attempt to take the EpiPens® and use them as weapons!

MEDICALERT® BRACELETS

A MedicAlert® bracelet is worn to alert emergency personnel about the wearer's medical conditions. You should purchase a MedicAlert® bracelet for your child and have him wear it at all times, "24/7." Do not allow him to remove it. Although he may object at first, eventually he will feel "naked" without it.

The MedicAlert® bracelet will be engraved with basic information about your child's condition (such as "Severely allergic to peanuts, dairy, egg").

More detailed information, including emergency contact names and phone numbers, your child's physicians, and information about any medication that she takes, will be stored on the MedicAlert® computers. In an emergency, emergency workers would be able to call MedicAlert® to access this potentially life-saving information.

———————

MedicAlert® bracelets are purchased from the MedicAlert Foundation. The MedicAlert Foundation's website is at www.medicalert.org. Contact information for their local offices in numerous countries is available through this site.

———————

Regardless of your child's age, he should wear a MedicAlert® bracelet. You may think that there is no need to purchase a MedicAlert® for an infant or toddler who is always with you. Think again. What if, for instance, you were incapacitated in an automobile accident and a well-meaning emergency worker tried to cheer up your uninjured milk- and peanut-allergic child with a peanut butter cookie and some milk? A severely food allergic infant or toddler should be wearing a MedicAlert® bracelet at all times.

———————

Periodically check your child's MedicAlert® bracelet for proper fit. When the bracelet starts to get too snug, order a larger chain. Your child's wrist will grow as she grows.

BE PREPARED

Keep your mobile phone charged, gasoline (petrol) in your car's tank, and some money in your wallet. Emergencies are never planned.

CHAPTER 2
TEACHING OTHERS ABOUT YOUR CHILD'S FOOD ALLERGIES

There are many adults who are a part of your child's life – including friends, relatives, neighbors, caregivers, teachers, coaches, and others – and it is a good idea to make all of them aware of your child's food allergies. Talk to these people. Tell them that your child has severe, potentially fatal food allergies. Tell them exactly what your child is allergic to and what they can do to help keep your child safe. If you will be leaving your child in their care, teach them how to recognize and treat an allergic reaction.

When teaching others about food allergies, you can share appropriate literature and educational videos. If available and appropriate, you can also share photographs of your child taken during a prior allergic reaction.

EXPECT DISBELIEF

Many people will find it hard to believe that "good, healthy foods" such as milk, bread, eggs and nuts can harm your child. They do not understand that for your child, one bite or less of an allergen really can lead to an extreme reaction or even death.

Be assertive in making your child's special needs clear. Remember, your child's life can be endangered by a well-meaning person who does not understand the importance of strict avoidance of allergenic foods.

HOW TO TEACH OTHERS TO RECOGNIZE AND TREAT ALLERGIC REACTIONS

Teachers, babysitters, friends, family members, scout leaders, sports coaches, carpool partners (school run partners), and others all need to know what precautions are necessary to keep your child safe, and what to do if your child has an allergic reaction while in their care.

To teach others how to recognize and treat your child's allergic reactions, start by putting the training information in writing. See Appendix B for a sample document.

Create a clear, typewritten document that explains:

❑ Exactly what your child is allergic to.

❑ Your child's common and possible symptoms during an allergic reaction.

❑ What to do during an allergic reaction, including how to administer an EpiPen® if one has been prescribed.

❑ When to call the rescue squad.

❑ Emergency contact information for you and other close relatives or friends.

❑ Name and phone number of your child's allergist.

❑ Your child's medical insurance information.

❑ If desired, attach a photograph of your child (this is especially useful if you will be giving the document to your child's school).

INTERNATIONAL PERSPECTIVE

COUNTRY	COMMENTS
United Kingdom	Medical insurance details would only apply for private insurance coverage. In the U.K., the NHS system treats anyone.

Special "EpiPen® Trainers" are available for teaching people how to use the EpiPen®. These "trainers" look like regular EpiPens® but do not contain a needle. As of this writing, in the U.S. a two-pack of EpiPens® comes with one free Trainer. Trainers are also available for purchase through the Food Allergy and Anaphylaxis Network (see Appendix A).

For each training session, you should:

❑ Give the trainee a copy of your written instructions.

❑ Go over all the details together, giving the person a chance to ask any questions.

❑ Show what your child's emergency medication looks like and where it is kept.

❑ For EpiPen® training, practice by using an EpiPen® Trainer.

❑ Continue the training session until the trainee feels comfortable and confident about responding to an allergic reaction.

WHEN OTHERS DON'T TAKE YOU SERIOUSLY

Dealing with adults who just don't "get it" can be very frustrating. Many people will think that you're exaggerating or are overly neurotic about the seriousness of your child's allergies. They do not believe that your child can die from a minor exposure to an allergen. However, this risk is real.

> *When Gay brought her severely nut-allergic daughter to a family gathering that was held in a community center room, she was incensed that one of her relatives had brought a nut dish to share. When confronted, this relative stated that she thought it would be okay to bring nuts because the party was not at Gay's house!*

There may be a number of reasons why a person just doesn't seem to "get it," including lack of education about food allergy, stress, fear, or simply not understanding what role is expected of him or her. The Food Allergy & Anaphylaxis Network (FAAN) has addressed this issue in their Food Allergy News newsletter[1]. FAAN recommends:

✦ Address problems as quickly as possible. Waiting to discuss a situation that occurred a month ago sends the message that what you have to say isn't urgent or important.

✦ Express your feelings and concerns in an open and honest manner, and allow others to do so as well.

✦ Avoid blaming and finger pointing. Use "I" and "we" statements, and watch your tone of voice.

✦ Identify the problem clearly. Ask the person for help in developing a solution that best suits everyone involved.

✦ Tell the person what you expect of him or her. Be specific, and keep requests reasonable.

✦ Educate the individual about food allergies. Offer published literature; some people find information more credible when it comes from various sources.

DO NOT ENDANGER YOUR CHILD

If, despite your best efforts, you still do not feel that a particular person understands your child's needs, do not leave your child in this person's care. Although this can be difficult (what if the person in question is your mother?), you must put your child's safety first.

---

[1] Food Allergy News Volume Twelve, Number One, page 5.

In spite of all of Erica and Dave's efforts to explain the seriousness of their daughter's allergy to their families (including sharing videos and written information explaining food-induced anaphylaxis), Dave's mo'' :r, a well-educated former nurse and head of outpatient services at a major hospital, refuses to believe that a food allergy can be life-threatening. She believes that Erica and Dave are fabricating the allergy in order to "control" their daughter Cherise.

When Cherise was a toddler, Grandma repeatedly tried to sneak Cherise the forbidden foods – even when Erica was at the house but had merely stepped out of the kitchen to use the restroom! When asked if she would only give Cherise foods that do not contain any allergenic ingredients, Grandma said, "No, I won't play that game." She has even gone so far as to state that Cherise will require "years of counseling" because of the "food controlling" which her parents are "imposing" on her! Sadly, Erica and Dave have had to forbid Dave's mother from ever being alone (even for a minute) with their daughter.

CHAPTER 3

GROCERY SHOPPING

Purchasing food for a child who has severe food allergies is not necessarily a simple matter, especially if your child is allergic to multiple items. Every item has to be scrutinized to determine if it contains the forbidden allergens.

Although at first it can be quite overwhelming, let me assure you that grocery shopping for your food-allergic child really will become relatively easy with practice. A lot of the hard work comes at the beginning, when you are first learning how to determine if a product is safe for your child, and you are first trying to find a selection of foods that your child can and will eat. After you get past this hurdle, it will all become second nature to you!

INGREDIENTS

Knowing exactly what is in the food which you feed to your child is one of the main keys to avoiding allergic reactions.

KNOW WHAT INGREDIENTS YOU MUST AVOID

Ask your child's allergist for a complete list of all the things that your child is allergic to and all of the ways that these items may be listed on an ingredient label. For example, "milk" may also be listed in numerous ways, including "casein," "whey," and "butter solids."

For a list of ways that the most common allergens may appear on an ingredient statement on foods sold in the United States, see Appendix C. Convenient wallet-sized "How to Read a Label" cards showing this information can be purchased from FAAN.

**INTERNATIONAL
PERSPECTIVE**

COUNTRY	COMMENTS
New Zealand	Ingredient Label Cards are also available for purchase from Allergy New Zealand. Go to www.allergy.org.nz to download the resource order form.

ALWAYS READ THE INGREDIENT STATEMENT

Do not rely on visual inspections of food items to determine whether or not a particular item is safe for your child! You cannot always tell what is in a food by looking at it, and allergens tend to turn up in the most unexpected places. For instance, many Thanksgiving turkeys are injected with a broth mixture that contains soy and milk ingredients. Would you have realized that raw turkey contains more than just "turkey"?

————————

You must check the ingredient statement of every item you purchase, every time you purchase it. Product ingredients may change without notice.

> *Once when my son was a toddler he and I went to the grocery store to do our weekly shopping. Upon arrival I grabbed a loaf of the brand and variety of bread that I purchased every week and handed him a slice. By the time I reached Aisle #2 Jason's face was bright red and breaking out in hives. Had I read the label on the bread before feeding it to Jason, I would have seen that the ingredients had changed and the bread now contained milk.*

————————

> *Barbara once purchased two apparently identical packages of chocolate chips. They were both the same brand, variety, and size. Barbara read the ingredient statement of the first package, and then bought them both. When she got the chocolate chips home she took a closer look and discovered that one package had a "may contain peanuts" statement...and the other did not!*

————————

If there is no ingredient statement available, do not let your child eat the food.

WHAT ARE "NATURAL FLAVORINGS" AND "ARTIFICIAL FLAVORINGS"?

Be aware that "natural flavorings" and "artificial flavorings" are catch-all terms that can refer to a wide variety of potentially allergenic ingredients. The only way to find out exactly what is in these "flavorings" in the product that you're evaluating is to contact the manufacturer.

 INTERNATIONAL PERSPECTIVE

COUNTRY	COMMENTS
Australia and New Zealand	As of Dec. 2002, peanuts, tree nuts, crustacea, fish, milk, gluten-containing cereals (wheat, rye, barley, oats, and spelt), eggs, soy bean and sesame seed must all be declared on the labels of packaged foods when present as an ingredient, part of a compound ingredient, a food additive or component thereof, or a processing aid or component thereof. Sulphites must be declared when present at a level greater than 10 mg/kg.

INGREDIENTS THAT SOUND LIKE MILK BUT ARE NOT

If your child is allergic to milk products, there are a number of common ingredients that sound like "milk" ingredients but actually are not. According to the Food Allergy and Anaphylaxis Network (FAAN), the following ingredients do not contain milk protein and need not be restricted by someone who has a milk allergy[1] :

✦ Calcium lactate

✦ Calcium stearoyl lactylate

✦ Cocoa butter (this is a derivative of the cocoa bean)

✦ Cream of tartar

✦ Lactic acid (however, lactic acid starter culture may contain milk)

✦ Oleoresin

✦ Sodium lactate

✦ Sodium stearoyl lactylate

---

[1] Reprinted with Permission from the Food Allergy and Anaphylaxis Network website, www.foodallergy.org.

INGREDIENTS THAT SOUND LIKE NUTS BUT ARE NOT

The following ingredients are not nuts, although they sound as though they are:

✦ Water chestnuts

✦ Nutmeg

———✦———

Coconut is the fruit of the palm, and is not generally considered to be a tree nut.

"NON-DAIRY" PRODUCTS MAY ACTUALLY CONTAIN DAIRY

As of this writing, the U.S. has no law regulating the use of the term "non-dairy" on product packaging. If your child is allergic to dairy products, keep in mind that foods labeled as "Non-Dairy" often are not non-dairy. For example, "non-dairy whipped topping" often contains casein, which is milk protein. Always check the ingredient statement carefully.

DIFFERENT VERSIONS OF PRODUCTS CAN HAVE DIFFERENT INGREDIENTS

"Low-fat" or "reduced-fat" versions of products sometimes contain different ingredients than "regular" versions. Always check the ingredient statement!

———✦———

"Snack size" versions of candy can contain different ingredients and/or be processed on different equipment than full size candies. Once again, always check the ingredient statement of every item you serve to your child, every time you buy or receive it.

———✦———

Different types of containers of the same product (i.e., shelf-stable carton vs. can) may contain different ingredients.

IMPORTED FOOD ITEMS

Be especially wary of imported packaged foods. Labeling laws and requirements vary by country. The labeling laws of the country from which the food was imported may be less rigorous or consistent than the laws of your country.

OTHER INGREDIENTS TO WATCH OUT FOR

✦ **Simplesse®**   If your child is allergic to dairy products or eggs, be aware
  Artificial   that Simplesse® artificial fat (used as an ingredient in
  Fat   potato chips, baked goods, and other products) is made
                    from dairy whey and egg protein.

✦ **Egg**   If your child is allergic to eggs, be aware that most com-
  Substitutes   mercial brands of liquid "egg substitutes" contain egg
                    whites. These products are designed for people who are
                    on a low-cholesterol diet, not for those who are on an
                    egg-free diet.

✦ **Liqueurs**   Although you are not likely to be serving your child li-
                    queur, be aware that many liqueurs are nut-based (such as
                    Amaretto, which is almond flavored). Watch out for can-
                    dies and desserts which contain liqueurs.

CHECK INGREDIENTS OF NON-FOOD ITEMS, TOO

In addition to checking the ingredient labels of all of the food that you
purchase, you also need to check the ingredients of lip balms, cosmetics,
soaps, skin care lotions, shampoos, ointments, and so forth. Don't assume
that these types of products will be free from ingredients to which your child
is allergic. I've seen a wide range of food products in shampoos (including
nut extracts and wheat), fish oil in lipstick, almond oil in soap, and olive oil
and cocoa butter in antibiotic ointment. Be careful, especially if the product
will go on the lips or in the mouth!

 **INTERNATIONAL
PERSPECTIVE**

COUNTRY	COMMENTS
United Kingdom	In the U.K., ingredients of cosmetics or personal care products may be listed on the package in Latin. A list of translations of common allergens is available from the Anaphylaxis Campaign, www.anaphylaxis.org.uk.

"Hypoallergenic" and "sensitive skin" cosmetics often contain
food ingredients. These products may not be "hypoallergenic" for your child.

Check the ingredients of the household cleaning products that you use, especially if citrus is a problem for your child.

————— ❧ —————

Although it is not common in the United States, many baby ointments commonly available in other countries contain peanut oil.

ALSO CHECK YOUR PET'S FOOD

Many pet foods contain ingredients to which your child may be allergic. I personally have seen peanuts and whey (a milk derivative) in bird seed, and egg in puppy food. If there is any chance that your child will be coming in contact with your pet's food (especially if you have a toddler who may decide to sample the pet's food or a puppy that may spread food throughout the house), you must be sure that this food is "hypo-allergenic" for your child.

THE PROBLEM OF
FOOD CROSS-CONTAMINATION

For most children with severe food allergies, cross-contamination is an important issue for you to address.

WHAT IS CROSS-CONTAMINATION?

Most food manufacturers use the same equipment to produce a variety of different products. Cross-contamination occurs when small amounts of residue from one product are still on the machinery when the next product is being produced. This results in minute amounts of the ingredients of product #1 ending up in product #2 – even though these ingredients will not be listed on the ingredient statement of product #2.

————— ❧ —————

Many – but not all – severely food-allergic children will react to foods which have been "contaminated" in this way. I am writing this book under the assumption that cross-contamination is a problem, but it is possible that this is not the case for your child.

"MAY CONTAIN" WARNINGS ON PRODUCT PACKAGING

Many food manufacturers do place warnings on the product box that the product "may contain traces of" an allergen or that it is "produced on machinery that also processes" allergens, or that it is "produced in a facility that processes" allergens. Because there is currently no standard of exactly what these designations mean, parents of severely food-allergic children are advised by FAAN to avoid any product which has one of these warnings regarding the allergens to which their child is allergic.

———— ◂❧▸ ————

"May Contain" warnings are usually placed near the ingredient statement, but are sometimes found in other locations on the product package. If there is no "May Contain"-type warning near the ingredient statement, you should also examine the rest of the package as well.

DOES A PARTICULAR PRODUCT HAVE A CROSS-CONTAMINATION RISK?

As of this writing, labeling laws in the U.S., Australia, Canada, New Zealand, and the U.K. do not **require** food manufacturers to warn consumers of possible cross-contamination. This labeling is completely voluntary. Therefore, the absence of a "may contain traces of X" notice does not necessarily mean that the food does not contain traces of X. The only way to be certain that a particular food is not produced on the same machinery as an allergen-containing product is to contact the food's manufacturer and ask.

———— ◂❧▸ ————

When trying to determine the likelihood that a particular product is produced on the same machinery as another, allergenic product, look to see if there are other flavors or varieties of the product in question – and then check the ingredients of those products. There is a good chance that all varieties of a given product are made on the same machinery.

CALL THE PRODUCT'S MANUFACTURER

If you have any doubts or questions whatsoever as to whether or not a particular product is safe for your child, contact the manufacturer to discuss the product's ingredients and the possibility of cross-contamination with other products. Do this before you feed the item to your child. See Appendix J for a sample "script" that you can use when contacting a food manufacturer to determine the safety of a particular product.

**INTERNATIONAL
PERSPECTIVE**

COUNTRY	COMMENTS
New Zealand	Allergy New Zealand has a guide for contacting food manufacturers, including sample forms for recording the information gathered, and a sample letter for sending to manufacturers.

Unfortunately, food manufacturer customer service personnel are not always knowledgeable about their company's manufacturing processes. Many parents of food-allergic children find that they can call the same company two times on the same day, speak to two different customer service representatives, ask the same questions, and get different answers regarding the safety of a particular product. For this reason, some parents choose to call the manufacturers of all of the foods which they wish to feed to their children multiple times (on different days) prior to letting their children ingest the food.

PERIODICALLY CALL THE MANUFACTURER AGAIN
Manufacturers can and do change their production processes without notice. You should regularly call the manufacturers of the foods which your child eats to verify that they are still safe.

> *When Gail's daughter Sara was 3 years old, the family walked down to the corner store to buy the "hypo-allergenic" frozen treat which Sara regularly ate. Sara took one bite and decided she did not want it. Her parents insisted she eat more, rather than wasting the expensive treat. Within minutes Sara was covered in hives, gasping for air, and experiencing a full-blown anaphylactic reaction. The next day Gail called the manufacturer and learned that the product was now made on shared equipment with a product that contained peanuts. The product label, however, did not reflect this fact.*

SIGN UP FOR FREE PRODUCT RECALL NOTIFICATION SERVICE
Even if you judiciously check ingredient statements and call manufacturers to grill them about their production processes, you can still never be sure

about packaged products. Errors regularly occur, and product recalls due to unlabeled allergens take place every week. To receive timely notices about many of these product recalls in the United States, visit www.foodallergy.org and sign up for FAAN's free product recall notification service.

 INTERNATIONAL PERSPECTIVE

COUNTRY	COMMENTS
Australia	Anaphylaxis Australia has a free product alert/recall notification service for members, and also lists this information on their website for general viewing. Visit their website, www.allergyfacts.org.au, for more information.
Canada	The Canadian Food Inspection Agency has a free product alert/recall notification service. Sign up at their website, www.inspection.gc.ca.
New Zealand	Allergy New Zealand has a free product alert/recall notification service. Sign up at www.allergy.org.nz.
United Kingdom	Details of product alerts are posted on the website of the Anaphylaxis Campaign, www.anaphylaxis.org.uk; details of the most serious alerts are mailed to members.

FOODS WITH HIGH RISK OF CROSS-CONTAMINATION

✦ **Nuts**   If your child is allergic to peanuts or tree nuts, it is usually best to avoid all nuts. Most peanuts and tree nuts are processed on shared equipment, and there is a very large risk of cross-contamination.

✦ **Chocolate Candies**   If your child is allergic to peanuts, tree nuts, or dairy products, be aware that most chocolate candies are produced on machinery that also processes nuts and dairy products. Unless you have contacted the product's manufacturer and verified that the product is safe for your child, it is best to avoid chocolate candies altogether.

✦ **Deli Counters**   Foods purchased at a deli counter have a particularly high risk of cross-contamination. Most delis use the same slicer for both meats and cheeses, making the meat unsafe for a milk-allergic individual (and vice-versa!). The prepared foods (such as egg-based potato salad, wheat-based pasta salads, and dishes containing nuts) may be dished up using a common utensil, so all of these dishes are unlikely to be safe as well.

✦ **Salad Bars** There is a high risk of cross-contamination at self-service salad bars, including those found in many grocery stores. Even if each salad item has its own serving utensil, customers often contaminate items by using a different item's utensil anyway. In addition, food pieces may fall from one bin into another while customers are serving themselves. For example, pieces of cheese may fall into the tomato bin, pasta may mix with the potato salad, and peanuts might end up in the dressing. I recommend that you avoid salad bars.

✦ **Bulk Items** Due to the very high chance of cross-contamination of food items, avoid all foods sold in bulk from barrels or other containers – i.e., the type of situation where you scoop up the desired quantity of unpackaged food (such as flour or oats or granola) and place it in a bag for pur-

✦ **Fresh Fish Counter** There is a high risk of cross-contamination between the various fresh fish and shell fish products available at the grocery store's fresh fish counter (where the various offerings are kept on display on ice and then wrapped up when purchased). If your child is allergic to any variety of fish or shell fish it is best to avoid all fish and shell fish that are sold in this way.

✦ **Nuts in the Produce Section** Watch out for open bins of nuts in the produce department. This can lead to nuts, nut particles, and nut "dust" contaminating everything around it. If this is the situation at your local store, talk to the store manager and see if he or she will agree to make some changes. If necessary, you may want to emphasize the risk that this poses for a segment of their customers, and make inferences to the legal liability that this implies for the store.

Julie went to her local grocery store (in South Carolina, the heart of "peanut country") and found an enormous bin of peanuts on display in the middle of the vegetable aisle. There were peanuts everywhere! The contamination was so widespread that it was not even safe for her young daughter to be there. Julie successfully spoke with the manager about the risk that these peanuts posed, and the bin of peanuts was removed.

KOSHER LABELING AND DAIRY ALLERGIES

Many parents of dairy-allergic children find it useful to check for the Kosher labeling of a product to help determine if the product contains dairy. "Kosher" foods are foods which meet Jewish dietary laws. These dietary laws prohibit the consumption of certain foods, require that foods be processed in certain ways, and, most importantly for the food allergic, prohibit the mixing of dairy products and meat products.

A basic explanation of Kosher labeling for the food allergic is as follows:

✦ In the Kosher system, foods are classified as being either "dairy," "meat," or "neutral" (neither dairy nor meat).

✦ Foods that meet the Kosher dietary laws are labeled with one of the Kosher symbols, including: K, ®, and Ⓤ. You can usually find these symbols in small type on the bottom front of the package.

✦ In the U.S., Kosher foods that contain dairy products usually contain a "D" or the word "Dairy" after the Kosher symbol.

✦ In the U.S., Kosher foods that are processed on Dairy equipment (i.e., equipment that is also used to process items which contain dairy) may have a "DE" after the Kosher symbol, although this is not always the case.

✦ In the U.S., Kosher foods that are considered neutral have the word "Pareve" or "Parve" after the Kosher symbol.

✦ In the U.S., The letter "P" in Kosher labeling never denotes "Pareve" – "P" designates "Kosher for Passover" (a Jewish holiday which has its own dietary laws).

✦ Not all foods are Kosher, and therefore not all foods contain a Kosher label.

**INTERNATIONAL
PERSPECTIVE**

COUNTRY	COMMENTS
Australia	In Australia, locally produced Kosher food is not marked with a symbol of any kind. A handbook called "The NSW Kosher Products & Services Directory" can be ordered from the NSW Kashrut Authority at www.ka.org.au; this book lists Australian Kosher products and explains the Kosher labeling system. According to this handbook, in Australia: • Kosher products that are considered "neutral" (i.e., Pareve) are marked with a "P" • Kosher products that contain dairy are marked with an "M" • Kosher products marked "P-DV" have been produced using dairy utensils.

Although the Kosher Dairy designation can be helpful for eliminating products, a severely dairy-allergic person cannot rely on the Kosher Pareve designation or the lack of a Kosher Dairy designation in determining the safety of a particular food. This is because it is possible for a food to contain a trace level of dairy contamination (something which might be a problem for your dairy-allergic child) and still be considered "Dairy-free" from the standpoint of the Jewish dietary laws. In other words, if the product is labeled as Kosher Dairy or Kosher Dairy Equipment, assume it contains dairy. In the absence of these labels, read the ingredient statement and take the same precautions that you would when evaluating any other product.

GOING TO THE GROCERY STORE

BRINGING YOUR FOOD-ALLERGIC CHILD TO THE GROCERY STORE

If you are taking your severely food-allergic toddler to the grocery store, be aware that she may react to food residue left on the grocery cart seat or handle by other toddlers. If this is a concern, prior to placing her in the grocery cart seat use wet wipes (which you bring with you from home) to clean the seat, handle, and other surfaces that she may touch.

FINDING DIFFICULT-TO-LOCATE ITEMS

If you do not live in a metropolitan area, you may find it difficult to locate some of the particular brands and varieties of foods which are safe for your child. Talk to the manager of your local grocery store; he or she may be happy to special order items for you. In addition, you can also pursue internet-based sources for special ingredients.

CONSIDER ONLY PURCHASING
"SAFE" PACKAGED GOODS FOR YOUR FAMILY

Consider only buying breads, crackers, potato chips, and other packaged foods for your household that are safe for your food-allergic child (even if the rest of the family is not on a restricted diet). This will cut down on errors and will avoid making your child feel left out.

If your child is allergic to milk products, consider only buying dairy-free margarine, and giving up butter completely. This will greatly reduce the chances of error when you cook. You will never have to ask yourself "Did I cook this with margarine or with butter?" and you will not need to worry about guests in your kitchen using the wrong spread when preparing your child's food.

NOTES

CHAPTER 4

FOOD IN YOUR HOME

I highly recommend that you make your home a "safe haven" for your child. Your home is one place where you should be able to relax and let your guard down a little. By creating a "safe haven" you will have the peace of mind associated with knowing that there are no allergenic foods within your young child's reach, and that there is no allergenic food residue hiding in your home.

It is important to note that studies have shown that the majority of food-allergic children will not experience anaphylaxis if they merely touch an allergen, although a localized reaction (such as hives) may occur. However, there is a real danger of a serious reaction if your child gets allergenic food residue on her fingers and then puts her fingers in her mouth, nose, or eyes, or touches and then consumes her otherwise "safe" food. Of course, even if your child initially only gets the allergen on, say, her leg, she may then get it on her fingers by scratching the hives that break out on her leg as a result of this contact. If your child is still at the age where she puts everything within reach into her mouth, this poses a further potential danger. By making your home a "safe haven," you minimize risks and create a more relaxing atmosphere for your family.

If your child is exquisitely sensitive, there is a chance that you may need to eliminate allergenic foods from your home entirely.

> *When she was about two years old, Gail's daughter Sara ate a tiny piece of food that she had found on the floor, tucked under the corner of the stove. Within minutes she suffered an anaphylactic reaction. After this terrifying experience Gail and her husband made the decision to eliminate all allergens from their home – despite the fact that Sara has multiple food allergies and a very limited diet.*

THE NEWLY DIAGNOSED SHOULD START WITH FRESH PACKAGES OF FOOD

If your child was just diagnosed with food-allergies, you should assume that all of the open packages of food in your home are "contaminated" with allergen. Chances are high that someone who had some sort of food residue on their fingers has stuck their hand into the box of crackers or bag of chips, there is peanut butter in the jam, bread crumbs in the butter, etc. Once you determine what is safe for your newly-diagnosed food-allergic child to eat, start with fresh packages of these items.

INTRODUCING NEW PRODUCTS TO YOUR CHILD

The **first time** that you feed your child a new product which appears to be safe (see Chapter 3 for a discussion of determining what products may be safe for your child), do not give her a full-size helping. Start with a tiny amount (possibly even a "lick"), and wait a little while to see if she reacts to it. Even if you have checked the ingredients and contacted the manufacturer, it is still better to take it slow. If the product turns out to be unsafe, your child's reaction to a small bite is likely to be less severe than a reaction to a full serving.

———❦———

Do not introduce more than one new food or new product per day. If your child has a delayed reaction to the food this will make it easier to determine exactly what caused the problem.

———❦———

Many children will undergo a period of "heightened reactivity" in the few days following an allergic reaction (even if it was a relatively minor allergic reaction). Therefore, if your child has had an allergic reaction in the past few days, now is not an appropriate time for her to try new foods or products.

———❦———

The best place to feed a new product to your child is at home – not the grocery store or the park or the family reunion! The best time to conduct a "new product test" is when you don't have anything else planned, and you will be available to monitor your child for an hour or so after she tries the food. Remember, a "new product test" is not an "allergen test." Tests to diagnose your child's allergies should **never** be done at home.

From experience I know that my son's reactions to food start almost immediately upon ingestion, usually within 1 minute. (Note: Your child's reaction time, of course, may be different than my son's, in which case you should adjust your "food test" accordingly). Whenever Jason tries a new food we start with what we call a "food test:"

1. *I take a good look at Jason's face and lips to be sure that he does not coincidentally have any hives or swelling prior to eating the food (and, now that he is a teenager, to note any pimples that I might later confuse with hives!).*

2. *I make sure that the medicine pack is handy.*

3. *Jason has a tiny bite of the food.*

4. *We set the kitchen timer for 3 minutes.*

5. *We sit and wait and see if anything happens.*

6. *When the timer rings I check Jason's face for signs of a reaction, and I ask him how his lips and tongue feel and how he feels in general.*

7. *During the test, the moment I see or Jason senses that anything is wrong, I give him a dose of his prescribed liquid antihistamine and then continue to watch him until he feels completely fine.*

This sort of thing is easier, of course, with an older child than it is with a baby or toddler!

CHILDREN OFTEN REFUSE TO EAT ALLERGENIC FOODS

It is interesting to note that children will often refuse to eat a food to which they are allergic – even if you and they are not aware of the allergy.

The blood test results for Anjali's daughter, Rebecca, showed very mild allergies to fish and corn, which the allergist did not think were serious. Anjali attempted to feed Rebecca a variety of different fish. Each time Rebecca would have a few bites, complain of an itchy throat, and state that she didn't care for the fish. Anjali stopped giving her fish for a year and a half and then re-introduced it, at which point Rebecca had a serious reaction that warranted a trip to the hospital. Rebecca does not like corn, either, so Anjali does not force her to eat it. "Perhaps," Anjali suggests, "the fact that she doesn't 'like' the food is her body's way of dealing with the allergies. It keeps her away from the food. My husband sometimes used to say, 'Anj, make her eat the corn,' but we have both decided now that we are not going to push her with any foods she really despises."

———— ❧ ————

I myself get violently ill if I eat beans. As a child my mother never made beans or anything which contained beans. I guess she simply didn't care for them. If beans were served when I was on a Girl Scout campout or spending the night at a friend's house, I would choose to go hungry rather than eat the beans. There was something about beans which I found repulsive, and I literally never tried them (not even one spoonful) until I was an adult – although as a child I would say that I "hated" beans. When I finally did try them, I learned that a few spoonfuls of beans will cause me to have an immediate and rather violent gastrointestinal response.

ALWAYS HAVE A SUPPLY OF "SAFE" FOOD AVAILABLE

Keep at least a few days' supply of "safe" food in your house. If you came down with the flu and couldn't get out, would you be able to feed your child? What if you could not leave the house due to inclement weather?

ALSO KEEP SOME PRE-COOKED "SAFE" FOOD ON HAND

It is a good idea to always keep at least one pre-cooked "safe" dinner in the freezer, to feed to your child on nights when you just do not have the time or energy to cook.

———— ❧ ————

It is also handy to keep safe cupcakes or other treats in your freezer, for your child to eat at birthday parties and other special occasions.

Every time Laura cooks something that can freeze – cakes, breads, ham, rolls, home-made pizzas, already-cooked French fries, you name it – she saves a serving to wrap up and put in the freezer. She keeps a special section of her freezer filled with cooked foods which she can grab as she's heading out the door.

In addition to keeping a supply of pre-made foods in her freezer, Laura also likes to keep a supply of frozen pre-cooked ground beef. Laura periodically prepares a large quantity of skillet-browned ground beef with chopped onions, and then repackages it into appropriate-sized freezer bags. She finds it convenient to use this meat as a base for quickly making spaghetti sauce, tacos and sloppy joes.

 INTERNATIONAL PERSPECTIVE

COUNTRY	COMMENTS
New Zealand	In New Zealand, "ground beef" is called mince.

IF YOU KEEP BOTH "SAFE" AND "NOT SAFE" FOODS IN YOUR HOME

Many people, especially parents of children who are only allergic to peanuts and/or tree nuts, choose to completely eliminate all allergenic foods from their home. Others, especially parents of children with multiple food allergies, do not make this choice. If for whatever reason you choose to keep both "safe" and "not safe" foods in your home, there are a number of issues which you must address and precautions which you must take.

LABEL FOODS IN YOUR HOME AS "SAFE" OR "NOT SAFE"

Many parents of young food-allergic children find it helpful to label all the food in their house as being either "safe" or "not safe." A convenient way to do this is to purchase a supply of red and green self-adhesive 1/2"- or 1"-diameter circle-shaped stickers from your local office supplies store. The red stickers are for the unsafe foods and the green are for the safe foods (i.e., "red" means "stop" and "green" means "go"). Apply these stickers to **every** item in your pantry, refrigerator and freezer.

———✱———

Every time you go grocery shopping, label every item purchased with the red or green stickers before you put it away. Your child will probably enjoy helping you with this. Although it takes effort to maintain, using this system allows your child – as well as babysitters, siblings, and others who visit your home – to easily determine which foods are safe and which are not.

AVOID MIX-UPS

If you keep both "safe" and "not safe" versions of similar items in your home (for example, soy milk and cow's milk, cheese-flavored crackers and dairy-free crackers), do not keep these products next to each other in the refrigerator or pantry. To avoid mix-ups, designate particular shelves or cabinets for storing the "safe" foods.

———————

If your milk-allergic toddler has non-allergic siblings, purchase a "special" sippy cup from which he is always served his beverages (both at home and away from home), and which is **never** used for anyone else. Put his name on it. Once you put the lid on the average sippy cup you cannot see the contents. Having a special cup that is always used ensures that your child doesn't grab the wrong cup by mistake.

AVOID CONTAMINATING
YOUR FOOD SUPPLY AND YOUR HOME

If you keep both allergenic and non-allergenic foods in your home, you need to ensure that the non-allergenic foods do not become contaminated through "casual contact." Teach all members of your household to wash their hands before touching the non-allergenic foods – even if they are touching it (during a meal or snack) in order to serve themselves. For example, your non-allergic daughter should not stick her allergen-covered hand into the box of crackers or bag of chips that are meant to be safe for her allergic sibling.

———————

Unless your entire household is on the exact same diet as your food-allergic child, you need to take precautions to ensure that your entire home does not become contaminated with allergenic food residue. Teach all members of your household to always wash their hands with soap immediately after eating or touching something allergenic. In addition, you may want to consider confining all food consumption to your kitchen and dining areas. Remember, if your husband eats dinner on the sofa and your daughter walks around the house eating snacks, crumbs and other residue are likely to find their way onto your carpets and furniture, and onto your children's toys.

———————

To facilitate all of this hand washing, keep a bottle of liquid hand soap and a roll of paper towels by your kitchen sink.

If you are going to allow your child's non-allergic siblings to eat allergenic foods in your home, do your best to teach them to eat neatly. Many children, especially young children, have a tendency to spread particles of food in a large radius about themselves when they eat. If these particles are allergenic, they can create a hazard for your food-allergic child, especially if these particles fall into the allergic child's food.

———————

To avoid having stray bits of dried allergenic food stick to your "clean" dishes, it is best to rinse off dirty dishes and utensils that are "contaminated" with allergenic foods prior to loading them into your dishwasher. Do this even if you have a high-quality dishwasher for which you do not normally pre-rinse your dishes.

———————

For a discussion of how to avoid cross-contamination while cooking, see Chapter 5.

LOCK YOUR REFRIGERATOR AND FOOD PANTRY

Until your child reaches an age at which you can trust him or her not to eat anything without your permission, keep childproof locks on your food pantry, refrigerator and freezer.

> *Samantha was taken by surprise when her sesame-allergic toddler got a hold of a jar of sesame seeds and rubbed them all over her face. Luckily she didn't actually eat any and her reaction was confined to some hives on her chin, but this did provide a "wake-up call" as to the need for locks on the family's food cupboard.*

UNEXPECTED FOOD INGREDIENTS IN NON-FOOD ITEMS

There are many non-food items in your home that are also potential sources of allergens. Watch out for:

✦ **Play Dough**   Commercially available "play dough" contains wheat. If your child is allergic to wheat, you can make a wheat-free homemade version. See Appendix L for sample recipe.

✦ **Bird Feeders**   If you keep a bird feeder in your yard, check the ingredients of the bird seed. Many commercially available bird seeds contain peanuts, wheat products, and milk products – plus, of course, seeds.

✦ **Stuffed**   Crushed and finely ground peanut or tree nut shells are
   Toys   sometimes used as part of the stuffing material of bean
                     bags, bean bag-type stuffed animals, "draft blockers" that
                     go under doors to prevent drafts, and other such items. If
                     your child is allergic to peanuts or tree nuts, only buy stuffed
                     toys and other items that are stuffed with polyester fiber-
                     fill or other synthetic products.

✦ **Pet Food**   As mentioned in Chapter 3, many pet foods contain
                     ingredients to which your child may be allergic. Watch
                     out for this in your home, and watch out for this when
                     visiting other people's homes.

✦ **Anything**   If your child is a baby or toddler, be especially careful of
   You Give   anything that you give to her to hold or play with. Babies
   to Your   and toddlers put everything into their mouths.
   Baby or   Anything given to them must be completely safe and free
   Toddler   of allergenic food residue.

*Joanne let her 13-month-old daughter play with the car keys,
and within minutes Elena's face swelled up. Evidently some
food residue had gone from Joanne's hand to the keys to
Elena's mouth.*

CHAPTER 5

COOKING

———————◆———————

Depending on the specifics of your child's allergies, cooking can be "no big deal" or a real challenge. If your child is only allergic to nuts, cooking everything "from scratch" is actually quite simple – just leave out the nuts. If you don't keep any nuts, nut oils, or products which contain or "may contain" nuts in the house, there will be nothing to worry about in the cooking department. If, however, your child is allergic to multiple items or to more-difficult-to-avoid items, you will need to find some new recipes and learn a new approach to cooking.

———————◆———————

As much as possible, I recommend you prepare food for your entire family which is also safe for your food-allergic child. Although some of your family may balk at the change in diet, keep in mind that it is an awful lot of work to cook two different menus for each meal. Depending on your allergic child's diet, it can be possible to eat wonderful food even on a limited diet.[1]

MENU PLANNING

Planning menus for a person with multiple food allergies can be a seemingly daunting task. Couple this with some children's natural fussiness, and many parents become understandably overwhelmed.

———————◆———————

Look for appropriate recipes in specialized cookbooks (such as mine!), newsletters, and on the internet. You may also find some suitable recipes in your existing recipe collection.

---

[1] For example, I wrote a cookbook, *What's to Eat? The Milk-Free, Egg-Free, Nut-Free Food Allergy Cookbook* (see order form at back of book) on the premise that "hypo-allergenic" food can be delicious, "normal," and easy-to-prepare.

Focus on what your child **can** eat instead of focusing on what your child **cannot** eat. For example, if your child is allergic to milk, eggs, and nuts, focus on serving delicious meals centered around grains, fruits and vegetables, legumes, fish, poultry and meats. Strive to find tasty and attractive alternatives so your child will not feel deprived.

AVOID CROSS-CONTAMINATION BETWEEN "SAFE" AND "UNSAFE" FOODS

Take steps to ensure that you do not contaminate your child's food with allergens during the cooking or serving process. Do not use the same utensils to simultaneously prepare allergenic and non-allergenic dishes.

———— ❧ ————

If you are preparing both allergenic and non-allergenic food for the same meal (such as sandwiches with or without mayonnaise and cheese), avoid cross-contamination in the preparation process by always preparing the non-allergenic meal first – before you even open the allergenic ingredients.

———— ❧ ————

If your child is allergic to ingredients that you regularly use in preparing food for other members of your household (such as wheat bread, cheese and mayonnaise), get in the habit of placing all contaminated utensils, plates, cutting boards, etc. directly into the sink or the dishwasher immediately after use. Teach your household that soiled items in the sink or dishwasher are not to be used again until they have been properly washed. This will help you avoid cross-contamination in preparing food for your allergic child, and will also help avoid contaminating your "safe" foods with allergenic particles that were left on the knife, cutting board, etc.

———— ❧ ————

Take precautions to ensure that your non-allergenic foods do not become contaminated by allergenic foods. For example: If a knife containing butter has been inserted into a jar of jam, this jam is no longer safe for a dairy-allergic individual to eat. If a knife is used to spread some butter on a piece of wheat bread, and the stick of butter is then touched by this now bread crumb-covered knife, the butter will not be safe for a wheat-allergic individual to eat.

———— ❧ ————

Mixing bowls, pots, pans, utensils, and so forth that have been used in the preparation of allergenic foods must be thoroughly washed in hot, sudsy water prior to being used to prepare food for your allergic child.

If you use your barbecue to cook both allergenic and non-allergenic foods, be sure to thoroughly clean the grill before cooking for your food-allergic child.

SERVING PEANUT BUTTER IN THE HOME OF A PEANUT-ALLERGIC CHILD

Because peanut allergy tends to be so severe – with allergic individuals reacting to minute quantities of peanut – most families of peanut-allergic children choose to completely ban all peanut products from their home. I highly recommend that you do this as well.

If your child is allergic to peanuts and you choose to serve peanut butter sandwiches to other members of your household, there are a number of precautions which you should take:

✦ Do not feed peanut butter to a child who is too young to eat it neatly (i.e., without it getting on his clothing and all over the table and chair).

✦ Do not touch peanut butter with your sponge. You will not be able to get all of the peanut butter particles out of the sponge.

✦ Use a plastic knife to spread the peanut butter and cut the sandwich, and then throw the knife away.

✦ Do not touch any other foods (such as the jam in your jam jar) with this knife.

✦ Make and serve the peanut butter sandwich on a paper plate, and dispose of the plate immediately after the meal.

✦ Thoroughly wash your hands with soap and water after preparing the sandwich.

✦ Ensure that the person who eats the sandwich thoroughly washes their hands (and face, if necessary) with soap and water as soon as they are finished eating – before they touch anything (including chairs, tables, and door knobs).

✦ Even if the sandwich is eaten away from home, the sandwich eater still must wash up immediately after eating…before the food gets on his clothing or he comes in contact with your car, your home, or your allergic child.

COOKING STUFFED POULTRY

If you are making poultry stuffing which contains ingredients to which your child is allergic, cook this stuffing in a separate dish – not in the bird. The proteins of the stuffing can be absorbed into the meat during the cooking process, making the meat unsafe for your child.

COOKING WITH DAIRY-FREE MARGARINE

If your child is allergic to milk, you will need to do some searching and taste-testing to find the best dairy-free margarine available in your area. A good margarine can make a big difference in many recipes, especially in baked goods. For baked goods, try to find a dairy-free margarine with a low water content (e.g., if you melt a stick of margarine, it should not be mostly water). Margarines with a high water content produce inferior baked goods.

SUBSTITUTING OTHER FLOURS FOR WHEAT FLOUR

There are a variety of "formulas" for substituting other flours for wheat flour in baked goods recipes. You may want to experiment to see what works best for you, given all of your child's allergies. I want to warn you, though, that alternative flours will not produce the same texture and consistency as wheat flour — in my opinion, the most you can hope for is a "pretty good" substitute. Possible 1-ingredient substitutes for 1 "measure" (such as 1 cup) of wheat flour include:

✦ 7/8 "measure" rice flour

✦ 1-1/3 "measure" ground rolled oats

✦ 1 "measure" corn flour

✦ 1 "measure" tapioca flour

———————✦———————

Some cooks feel they get better results when they mix together a few different flours. Some multi-ingredient wheat flour substitution formulas are:

✦ 4 parts oat flour + 2 parts barley flour + 1 part rice flour

✦ 1 part rye flour + 1 part potato flour

✦ 1 part cornstarch + 2 parts rice flour + 2 parts soy flour + 3 parts potato starch flour

> *Barbara likes to keep a container of pre-mixed flour in her pantry, so it is always ready and available when she needs it.*

EGG SUBSTITUTES FOR BAKED GOODS

There is no "egg-free egg substitute" for making eggs (i.e., scrambled eggs, omelets, fried eggs, etc.). However, it is possible to substitute for eggs in many baked goods recipes. My favorite egg substitution formula, which I use in most of the baked goods recipes in my "What's to Eat?" food allergy cookbook, is the combination of baking powder, vegetable oil and water which FAAN has been recommending for many years:

✦ To substitute for one egg in a baked goods recipe, use 1-1/2 tablespoons vegetable oil mixed with 1-1/2 tablespoons water and 1 teaspoon baking powder.

✦ To substitute for two eggs in a baked goods recipe, use 3 tablespoons vegetable oil mixed with 3 tablespoons water and 1-1/2 teaspoons baking powder.

✦ If a recipe for baked goods calls for 3 or more eggs per batch (with a typical "batch" consisting of 36 cookies, one pan of brownies, one loaf of bread, or one cake), it is my experience that egg substitutes do not work. The consistency of the finished product comes out poorly. Pound cakes, sponge cakes, angel food cakes, brownies, and other popular desserts with relatively high egg content do not turn out well in egg-free cooking. Rather than wasting your time and ingredients trying to create egg-free versions of these desserts, I recommend that you make something else instead!

SERVING COLD FOOD

Something you can do while your child is young that will really pay off for years to come is to get her accustomed to enjoying a variety of foods served either cold or at room temperature. Unless your child outgrows her allergies, you are likely to be bringing "special" food for her to social events, outings, vacations, and so forth for many years. It's a real convenience in these situations to have a child who will happily eat cold food straight out of the ice chest.

WHY YOU SHOULD TEACH OTHERS
HOW TO PREPARE FOOD FOR YOUR CHILD

After you learn all the "ins and outs" of purchasing and preparing food for your child, it is important that you teach all of this information to 1 or 2 close friends or relatives as well. In an emergency, there must be someone outside of your household who is capable of caring for your child. Of course, these people also need to be trained in the emergency procedures to follow in case your child has an allergic reaction while in their care (see chapter 2).

A few months after I published my What's to Eat? *food allergy cookbook I received an urgent e-mail from a woman on the East Coast. Could I please ship a copy to her via overnight express? The unthinkable had happened. Her sister-in-law had suffered a heart attack and was in a coma. Her brother was holding a bedside vigil at the hospital. Martha had rushed in to care for her 3-year-old food-allergic niece and her 5-year-old nephew.*

Although she knew that Grace was highly allergic to milk, eggs, and peanuts, Martha did not know how to read an ingredient statement to check for these items, how to avoid cross-contamination in the cooking process, or exactly what foods were safe. And she did not have or know how to use Grace's EpiPen®. The previous evening Grace had suffered an allergic reaction and had to be rushed to the hospital. The extended family's lack of detailed knowledge about how to care for Grace had made an incredibly difficult situation even worse.

Thankfully, Grace's story did have a happy ending. I e-mailed some basic instructions to Martha that day and had the book in her hands the next morning; Grace's extended family then had the tools to keep her safe. After 12 days in a coma Grace's mother woke up. The last I heard, her prognosis was excellent.

Regardless of the happy ending, you do not ever want your child to be in a situation such as this. Make sure that someone outside of your home can care for your child in an emergency.

CHAPTER 6

PARENTING

As a parent, you should strive to make it possible for your child to experience all of the typical activities of childhood. Your child should be able to go to school, have friends, participate in extracurricular activities, attend parties, go to camp, and so forth. Although many activities will require advance planning and preparation on your part, they are all possible.

EMOTIONS

Keep in mind that it is normal to occasionally feel jealous of your friends' healthy children and "normal" life. It is also normal to go through a "grieving" period when your child is initially diagnosed and again each time there is a significant (negative) development in your child's condition. Don't try to deny these feelings, but don't let them overwhelm you for very long, either. Stay focused on the positive, and know that you can keep your child safe and help him or her to grow up to be a healthy, well-adjusted adult. If these feelings do overwhelm you, seek help from a qualified professional.

Although caring for a child with life-threatening food allergies can be challenging, try to keep things in perspective. Avoid driving yourself crazy by obsessing on the "what ifs." Do your best to let go of the anxiety. Accept the fact that – just like in the rest of life – you can minimize the risks but you can never completely eliminate them. Yes, you need to be careful, take appropriate precautions, and be prepared for an emergency. But you should also keep in mind that prompt emergency treatment does indeed save lives, and because of this the actual number of food allergy deaths is relatively small.

GET INVOLVED

While your child is young, volunteer to be classroom parent, team parent or coach, scout leader, etc. You'll always be present in an emergency, and you will be in a position to minimize the chances that an emergency will happen at all.

TODDLERS

Any time you take your food-allergic toddler anywhere (including parks, playgrounds, other people's homes, grocery stores, shopping malls, parties, amusement parks, etc.) you need to stay within an arm's length distance of her, in order to prevent her from putting allergenic tidbits into her mouth.

TEACHING YOUR YOUNG CHILD ABOUT FOOD ALLERGIES

One of your goals as a parent needs to be to teach your child to take an active part in managing his or her food allergies. Here are some of the things which you should teach to your young food-allergic child...

FOOD ALLERGIES CAN MAKE YOU SICK

From a very early age (such as when you get the initial diagnosis), start teaching your child that he has food allergies and that if he eats something he is allergic to he can get very, very sick.

ONLY EAT OR TOUCH FOOD THAT MOMMY OR DADDY HAS APPROVED

Explain to your child that you're counting on him to help you by not eating **anything** unless you (or whatever other adults you have authorized to make these decisions) have checked the ingredients and say that the food is safe.

> *After her son Evan was diagnosed with food allergies, Janet got into the habit of always saying "Mommy has to check the ingredients" before handing her son anything to eat. When Evan started speaking, everyone got a good laugh when one of his first vocabulary words turned out to be "ingredients!"*

Teach your child not to so much as touch a food unless you (or whatever other adults you have authorized to make these decisions) have personally approved it. Even adults that your child knows (such as teachers and friends' parents) may not be able to tell if a food is safe. For example, while your child's teacher can certainly read the ingredient statement on a snack to see if egg is listed, she is not likely to know if that product has cross-contamination production line issues with another product (which you are familiar with because of your conversations with the manufacturer) or if it was recently recalled due to undeclared allergen (which you are aware of because you signed up for FAAN's free product recall notification service – see page 40).

DON'T TAKE FOOD FROM STRANGERS

Just as it is important to teach your child not to talk to strangers, you must also teach him not to take food from strangers – even if the "stranger" is a friendly mother at the park or at a birthday party.

> *Children can learn these lessons at a surprisingly young age. When Jake was 2 years old, he and his mother were at a birthday party. Barbara had turned her back to pour juice for another child when another mother offered Jake a slice of pizza. Barbara was surprised (and pleased) to hear him say, "I can't eat that. I'm allergic."*

SPEAK UP IF YOU DON'T FEEL RIGHT

As soon as your child is old enough to comprehend, teach her that if she ever feels sick, wrong, strange, or "funny" after or while she is eating something – such as if she is itchy or nauseous, she is having problems breathing, her lips or tongue are tingling, or she is inexplicably frightened – she needs to immediately tell you or the adult in charge about what she is feeling.

WASH YOUR HANDS BEFORE YOU EAT

As soon as your child is old enough to feed himself, start teaching him to always wash his hands before and after he eats.

WHAT ARE THE FOODS THAT YOU DO EAT CALLED?

Teach your child the real names for the "substitute" foods which he eats, such as "soy milk" and "margarine" instead of "milk" and "butter." Otherwise he may not realize that he is allergic to the "real" products.

WHEN IN DOUBT, SPIT IT OUT

Teach your child that if he ever accidentally takes a bite or a sip of something that he suspects he is allergic to, he should immediately spit it out. Tell him not to worry about being rude or disgusting, and not to wait until he can politely run to a sink or toilet. Teach your child: "when in doubt, spit it out!" This applies no matter what type of social situation your child may be in at the time.

When she was young, Marlee was served a supposedly "plain" bagel at a bagel shop. She took one bite, realized something was wrong, and immediately spit it out. This act, although probably perceived as exceptionally rude by the diners at the surrounding tables, may have saved her life. The underside of the "plain" bagel was covered with cream cheese.

WHAT DO ALLERGENIC FOODS LOOK LIKE?

When your child is a toddler, start teaching her what the allergenic foods look like. After all, if you do not keep the offending foods in your home, she may not even be able to recognize them. Show her pictures of the foods. Point out allergenic items in the grocery store, in advertisements, in picture books, and on television. Your peanut-allergic child, for instance, should know what a peanut looks like.

You can start this education when your child is quite young. When Ann's son Beau was only 18 months old, he could already recognize pictures of things he could not eat.

———◣✦◢———

This is something which I did not do a sufficiently thorough job of myself. When Jason was in first grade, he attended a school which had a focus on hands-on learning materials. Although the teacher, Mr. Alex, had meticulously gone through all of the materials to remove any "hazardous" items (and had then washed everything that these items had come in contact with), he missed one. His heart must have stopped when he heard Jason say, "Mr. Alex, what's this?" and turned to see Jason holding up the chestnut that he found in the "ch" phonics container.

WHAT IS AN EPIPEN®?

Explain to your child that the EpiPen® is a very special medicine that you always carry with you in case she has an allergic reaction. Explain to her that in this situation, the EpiPen® is a medicine that will make her feel better right away.

———◣✦◢———

Use the EpiPen® trainer with your child, to try to decrease any mystery or fear that may be associated with the EpiPen®.

When your child is preschool-age, you can buy her a toy "doctor's kit," and add the EpiPen® trainer as another "doctor thing" for her to play with. However, you do need to make it clear that the real EpiPen® contains real medicine (and a needle) and is therefore not a toy.

TEACHING AN OLDER CHILD ABOUT FOOD ALLERGIES

As your child gets older you should continue to teach her about food allergies in an age-appropriate way, as well as get her increasingly involved in managing her allergies.

RECOGNIZING NAMES OF ALLERGENIC INGREDIENTS

When your child is somewhere between the ages of 4 and 6 you can start to teach her to recognize the names of all the ingredients to which she is allergic (such as "casein" and "whey" for a child who is allergic to dairy products). Read labels out loud to your child. Make it a game to see if your child can recognize the name of the allergen when she listens to you read an ingredient list. See Appendix C for a list of ways that common ingredients may be shown on an ingredient statement.

However, **never** give your young child the responsibility of determining whether or not a given food is safe for her to eat. Until your child is much older, this must be the responsibility of an adult.

WHAT IS CROSS-CONTAMINATION?

When your child is old enough to understand, teach her about the concept of "cross-contamination" – that foods which would usually be safe for her can become "contaminated" with allergens during the cooking process, at the manufacturing plant, or through casual contact with the allergen. When she understands this, she will understand why it may not be safe to eat food that was prepared in a friend's kitchen, and why it may not be safe to eat normally "safe" foods (such as jam) when at someone else's house.

CREATE A SPECIAL "DISTRESS" SIGNAL

As your child gets older, you may wish to create a special signal or secret word that he can use to let you know that he is having a reaction. Many children are reluctant to call attention to themselves, especially in a public place or a social gathering. A signal may be a more comfortable way for your child to let you know that something is wrong.

PRAISE POSITIVE BEHAVIOR

Look for opportunities to reinforce your child's positive behavior. Complement him when he turns down allergenic food, tells you he isn't feeling right, reads the label, recognizes allergens, etc.

WOE IS ME

At some point, your child is likely to decide that being "special" just isn't that "special" anymore. What do you do when your food-allergic child becomes unhappy with her lot in life and begins to complain about her allergies and the impact that they have on her life? Assuming the problem is not so great as to require professional intervention, the best thing to do is to offer a sympathetic ear and listen. Encourage your child to express her emotions. Once she has let it out, you can agree with her that having allergies is not "fair." However, you also need to emphasize that this is the way it is, you cannot change the situation, and you need to work together to make the most of it. Life isn't fair. If you think it would be helpful, you can also point out others in your child's life that have "differences" or medical challenges.

If you belong to a food allergy support group, you can arrange for your child to have a heart-to-heart talk with another child of similar age who is coping well. The other child may be able to help your child put things in a positive light.

FOOD ALLERGIES CAN BE FATAL

At some point you will need to explain to your child that not only can he get "very very sick" if he eats the wrong thing, but the reaction can be potentially fatal. This is a horrible thing to have to tell your child. What is the appropriate age at which to bring this up? This varies greatly for each child. Some of my friends explained this when their children were as young as 5, others wait until their child is 9 or 10. Whenever you do feel it's the right time to share this information with your child, this conversation is the time to emphasize to your child that every day you do everything you can to keep him safe (including checking ingredient labels, carrying his medication, and always being sure that there is a responsible and trained adult available in case of an emergency), and to tell him how proud you are of his cooperation in these efforts.

DEALING WITH AN UNCOOPERATIVE CHILD

As your child gets older, he may start to become tempted to try foods while he is away from you (such as a bite of his friend's lunchbox cookie or a taste of another pal's cafeteria lunch). He may believe that he can "recognize" safe foods, or he may have an urge to try the "forbidden" foods that everyone else raves about. You will have to work with him to get him to understand how dangerous this behavior is.

Years ago I was mortified to learn that while on a class whale-watching excursion (on a boat, two hours from shore), my son ate quite a few of his friend's saltine crackers. The crackers were in an unmarked plastic bag, but they "looked just like the ones that we have at home." As it turns out, they evidently were the same brand we buy at home, but that didn't lessen my concerns about what could have happened. I had sent him off on this field trip feeling completely confident that he would never take food from someone else... but he did.

For a child, the vague concept of getting very ill – or the even more esoteric concept of death – may not be much of a deterrent to dangerous food-eating behavior. If your child is exhibiting dangerous behavior, and your talks with her are not having any affect on the behavior, you may need to frighten her with a fairly graphic description of what could happen during an anaphylactic reaction. Although you can mention the possibility of hives, swelling, and the inability to breathe, it may be more effective to discuss the possibility of her losing control of her bowels in front of all of her friends. For most school-age children, this thought will be a powerful deterrent to dangerous behavior.

ROLE PLAY

Role play with your child. Depending on your child's age, practice how to handle some of the situations that are likely to come up, such as:

+ Being offered food by an adult
+ Having different food than other guests at a party
+ Peer pressure to try new foods or to trade food
+ Teasing
+ Harassment
+ Questions about your child's allergies, diet, MedicAlert® bracelet, fanny pack, etc.
+ Situations where other children have visible (possibly allergenic) food on them, such as on the school playground after lunch
+ Situations where the play equipment has visible food residue on it

FURTHER IDEAS FOR OLDER CHILDREN

For further ideas regarding teaching your child about food allergies, and preparing him to eventually manage his own food allergies, I recommend FAAN's booklet, "Letting Go: Teaching a Child Responsibility," or the (U.K.) Anaphylaxis Campaign's similar booklet, "Letting Go: Teaching an Allergic Child Responsibility." Visit the appropriate organization's website for ordering information.

WORKING WITH YOUR TEEN OR PRE-TEEN

As your child moves on to the teen years you will have to develop new methods for managing his food allergies. Your child will want and need greater independence. At school you will probably move from a situation in which all of your child's classmates are educated about his food allergies to a situation where your child's classmates are only informed on a "need-to-know" basis. Letting go can be very stressful.

GENERAL TIPS

On their website and in the Food Allergy News newsletter, FAAN has provided these tips for coping with this new stage in your child's life[1]:

✦ Recognize that new rules will be needed at each stage of your child's development (i.e., as they advance in grades) and plan for them before you need them.

✦ Help your child develop a plan that suits everyone. Allow your child to have input. How will after school activities be handled? Talk about dances, football games, where to eat, how to store medications, sources of "safe" foods, and how to handle unexpected situations and reactions.

✦ Outline what responsibilities your child will now take on. If necessary, write them down as a formal agreement. What are the consequences of not following the agreement?

✦ Discuss who will need to know about the food allergy; i.e., each time your child leaves the house with a group of friends, at least one of them should be familiar with the food allergy, and know what to do in the event of a reaction.

✦ Empower your child. Use messages such as, "I trust you," and "You can do this," rather than "You can't," or "How do you expect to…"

✦ Try not to nag excessively. Gentle persuasion, such as "Are you sure you have your EpiPen® with you?" or "Please be sure to check with the

---

[1] *Food Allergy Newsletter* Volume Eleven, Number Six, August-September 2002, page 1-2, and FAAN Website, www.foodallergy.org, *"The Adolescent and Food Allergy: Survival Tips for Parent and Child,"* by Dr. Bob Wood.

manager before you order," would be appropriate reminders before your teenager goes out for the evening.

✦ If your teenager is refusing to take the necessary precautions to safeguard his health (including strict avoidance of allergens and carrying his emergency medication at all times), it may be best to enlist the help of your child's allergist in communicating with your child.

———— ✧ ————

For additional tips from FAAN, I recommend you order their "Learning to Live With Food Allergies: Tips for Parents and Teens" two-booklet set. This set comes with one booklet for the parent and one for the teen. The "teen" book addresses commonly asked questions and provides some tips for minimizing risks, all in age-appropriate language. You can order the booklets at www.foodallergy.org.

GOURMET COFFEE SHOPS

Gourmet coffee shops are popular teenage hang-outs. If your teen has a nut or egg allergy, however, beware. Many gourmet coffee flavors include nuts (such as "Hazelnut Roast"); even in the "plain" flavors, there is a high risk of cross-contamination. In addition, egg is sometimes used to create the foam topping on specialty coffee drinks. A safer alternative would be to order tea.

DRUGS AND ALCOHOL

When you speak to your teen about the dangers of alcohol and drugs, explain that these substances pose an additional risk to the food-allergic: Alcohol and drugs will impair his judgment, thereby increasing the chances that he will eat an allergenic food or not notice when a reaction is starting.

KISSING

Make sure that your teen understands that a reaction can occur from kissing someone who recently has eaten food to which he is allergic. Once your child begins dating, he should not attempt to "hide" his food allergies from the people with whom he goes out. He needs to be honest and upfront, and enlist his date's help in keeping him safe.

ATTENDING CATERED EVENTS

At some point in time, your teen or pre-teen may be invited to a formal catered social event, such as a wedding or Bar Mitzvah. In these cases, I recommend that your child bring his own food. Even if you were to call the caterer in advance to discuss ingredients, food preparation methods, and so forth, the risk of some last-minute change being made – or the food becoming cross-contaminated with something being prepared for a different party – is very high.

———— ❧ ————

If your child will not be eating the food provided, you should make the host aware of this fact at the time that you send in your R.S.V.P. Most caterers charge by the person. Your host should not have to pay for a plate of food that your child cannot eat.

———— ❧ ————

You and your child need to decide in advance whether or not he will eat **any** of the food being served, including something which appears "safe." My advice is that he only eats the food brought from home, especially if he will be attending the party on his own.

———— ❧ ————

Prior to the day of the event, talk to your child about the etiquette of bringing food to a catered event.

> *It didn't occur to my 12-year-old son that it would not be appropriate at a nice catered luncheon for him to set his lunchbox on the table and eat directly out of it (like he would at school). I instructed him to obtain a clean plate from the wait staff or buffet line, take the food out of the containers we packed it in and place it on the plate, place the empty food containers back into the lunchbox, and then place the lunchbox under his seat.*

———— ❧ ————

If your daughter is not comfortable bringing a lunchbox or bag to a formal event, she can bring it in a large, stylish purse.

———— ❧ ————

If your child is severely allergic to nuts, you may want to call the hostess in advance to inquire if there will be dishes of nuts set out at the tables or if there will be nuts used in the centerpieces (such as peanuts in a "baseball"-themed display). If the answer is yes, you need to assess whether or not it will be safe for your child to attend the event.

———— ❧ ————

As usual, make sure that your child carries her medicine kit with her at all times.

OTHER FAMILY MEMBERS

Your entire household will be affected by your child's food allergies.

SIBLINGS

Your child's non-allergenic siblings may resent the extra attention that is focused on the allergic child, or may complain about the "unfairness" of the activities in which your family cannot participate or the foods that your family does not serve because of their sibling's special needs. If possible, try to make regular arrangements for you, your spouse, or another close adult friend or family member to take the other children out of the house to eat these foods and enjoy these experiences.

When my son Jason is spending some time at a friend's home, his brother Kevin and I usually go straight to the donut shop. If Kevin and I are alone together during a mealtime, we often head for the local Chinese buffet or "soup and salad bar" restaurant.

If the non-allergic sibling is still young enough to make a mess of himself when eating, you will need to take precautions after these food outings to avoid contaminating your car and your house with allergens.

When Donna's husband takes their young non-allergic daughter out to breakfast, he brings along a complete change of clothing for her to put on before coming home. When Kevin & I go out for donuts, we clean our hands prior to returning to the car.

Although you can and should lend a sympathetic ear when your non-allergic children feel a need to complain about the situation, make it clear that it is not acceptable for them to complain to or tease their food-allergic sibling. Your home should be a place of love and understanding, where each member of the family, including the food-allergic child, is accepted as he is.

SPOUSES

It often happens that spouses have very different styles of dealing with their child's food allergies, and this can easily become a source of strife.

Anjali says, "My husband likes to take 'risks' in all aspects of his life. I, on the other hand, like to take 'no' risks. So, we carry this philosophy forward into how we manage Rebecca's allergies. I frequently have to convince my husband that we cannot do something or we cannot eat something. Ultimately,

I feel that if we can do it my way without causing him any 'major grief' – and if doing it my way will make me feel tremendously more comfortable – then why can't we take my more conservative approach?"

———❧———

If your spouse is in denial about the seriousness of your child's allergies – and, as a consequence, is taking risks that could jeopardize your child's health – you will need to find a way to get through to him or her. Enlist the help of your child's allergist. Urge your spouse to read or view appropriate literature (such as this book), websites, and videos. Just as with any other caregiver who doesn't "get it," your child's life could be at stake.

———❧———

On the other hand, it could be that your spouse does have a full understanding of the seriousness of your child's allergies and does take appropriate precautions, but simply has a different style and approach than you do. In this case, this is a marital issue which the two of you need to negotiate. If this becomes an on-going marital problem, do not hesitate to seek help from a neutral third party, such as a qualified marital counselor. Caring for a child with life-threatening food allergies can be very stressful. Don't let this stress destroy your marriage.

HIRING A BABYSITTER

If you have created a safe home environment, it is possible to hire a babysitter so that you can go out. In fact, with the stress of caring for a "special needs" child, you probably need this respite more than the "average" parent does! However, like everything else in your life now, hiring a sitter requires extra planning.

HIRE A RESPONSIBLE, MATURE, EXPERIENCED SITTER

Although many of your friends may use "very responsible" sitters who are only 12 or 13 years old, you will probably want to employ sitters who are at least a little bit older and more mature than this. A level-headed 16-year-old would be better suited to the task. A college student or adult would be even better.

Your babysitter should have prior experience watching children of this age. Although you will need to teach her about your child's food allergies, she should already be a responsible and competent baby sitter.

HAVE THE SITTER COME TO YOUR HOME

Have the sitter watch your child in **your** home. You will have the piece of mind of knowing they are in as safe an environment as possible.

TEACH THE SITTER ABOUT
YOUR CHILD'S FOOD ALLERGIES

Pay the sitter to come over for an hour or two prior to the day when she will be staying alone with your children for the first time. Use this time for you and your children to get to know her, and to go over all of the emergency training. You should do the following:

❏ Have the sitter read your written emergency instructions (see pages 29-30).

❏ Discuss your written emergency instructions in detail.

❏ Have the sitter practice using the EpiPen® by using an EpiPen® trainer.

❏ Show the sitter what your emergency medicine pack looks like and where it is kept.

❏ Show the sitter where you keep your emergency contact information. Make sure that this information includes the number for your mobile phone or beeper (if you have one) as well as the names and phone numbers of nearby friends and neighbors who are willing to be called if needed.

❏ Show the sitter the script for calling the rescue squad that you keep by the phone (see Appendix K).

❏ Show the sitter where all of your regular first aid supplies are kept.

❏ Explain to the sitter that she cannot bring ANY food into your home. If she gets hungry, she can help herself to the "safe" food that is in the house.

❏ Ask the sitter to wash her hands with soap just prior to coming over to your home.

FEED YOUR CHILDREN BEFORE YOU LEAVE

Plan to either feed your children dinner before you leave, or prepare a completely safe home-cooked meal that the sitter will serve and eat with your children.

ON THE DAY YOU GO OUT

On the day that you go out, have the sitter arrive at least 20 minutes before you need to leave. Use this time to:

❏ Review the emergency instructions with the sitter one more time.

❏ Show the sitter where you have left a signed "Authorization to Consent To Treatment of Minor" form (see Appendix F for a sample).

❏ Remind the sitter where the emergency medication is kept.

❏ Show the sitter exactly which foods can be consumed while she is there – both by the children and by her.

❏ Ask the sitter if she has brought any food with her. If she forgot your previous instructions and did bring food with her, take this food with you and give it back to her when you return!

❏ Don't forget to discuss all of the "normal" information that parents usually discuss with a sitter (such as bedtime routines, what time you plan to return, etc.)!

GIVE A POP QUIZ

Once someone becomes your "regular babysitter," you should periodically give her a food allergy "pop quiz" with questions such as "show me how to use the EpiPen®," and "when should you call the rescue squad?" You should do this in a non-threatening manner, emphasizing that you just want to keep the information fresh in her mind. Review the training information as necessary.

CARRY YOUR MOBILE PHONE WITH YOU

While you are gone, be sure to carry your (fully-charged) mobile phone or beeper with you...and make sure that it is turned on and set to ring!

WHEN YOU RETURN HOME

When you return, talk to the sitter to see how things went and how comfortable she was caring for your food-allergic child. If things went well, make plans to go out again!

FOOD ALLERGIES AND HOLIDAY CELEBRATIONS

Most holiday celebrations revolve around food. Chances are you will find that most of this food cannot be eaten by your child. So what can you do to ensure that holidays are a source of joy and happiness for your child anyway?

DE-EMPHASIZE FOOD

For one thing, do whatever you can to take the emphasis away from the food. Focus your child's attention on the happiness of being with family and friends, on the festiveness of the occasion, on the non-food activities, and (if appropriate) on the gifts.

ATTENDING HOLIDAY PARTIES

From the perspective of creating a safe environment for your child, holiday parties (Christmas parties, Thanksgiving dinners, Easter brunches, and so forth) are just like any other social occasion. See Chapter 7 for a lengthy discussion of attending social events.

If your child will not be able to eat the food which is being served, make a special effort to bring some of her favorite foods for her to eat at the party. It is depressing to eat something boring (or, worse, unappealing) while everyone around you is raving about the fabulous holiday delicacies.

HOSTING HOLIDAY PARTIES

If it is possible for you to host the get-together at your house – with you committing to preparing all of the food yourself – it may be possible to create an entire hypo-allergenic holiday meal. For a milk-, egg-, and nut-free diet, for example, my book, *What's to Eat? The Milk-Free, Egg-Free, Nut-Free Food Allergy Cookbook* (see order form at back of this book), provides recipes for a complete holiday meal.

CHRISTMAS STOCKINGS AND ADVENT CALENDARS

Don't forget that Christmas stockings are often filled with candies, and Advent Calendars frequently contain imported chocolates or other treats. Be sure to purchase safe alternatives for your child.

PHOTOS WITH SANTA CLAUS OR THE EASTER BUNNY

If you are planning to take your child to the local shopping mall to have her picture taken with "Santa Claus" or the "Easter Bunny," be aware that some Santas and Easter Bunnies routinely give out candy. Bring a safe substitute in case this occurs.

EASTER BASKETS

Creating a safe Easter celebration for your food-allergic child can be a challenge. Brightly colored Easter eggs… Easter baskets filled with goodies….milk chocolate Easter bunnies. All of these things may pose a danger to your child. Suggestions for creating "safe" Easter baskets include:

✦ Substitute plastic eggs for real eggs; decorate with stickers, markers, lace, and other craft items.

✦ Use "safe" candy or "safe" non-candy food items (such as pretzels, fruit rolls, or fresh fruit).

✦ Fill plastic eggs with little trinkets, such as colorful erasers, stickers, jewelry, coins. Or use other non-food items, including trading cards, toy cars, chalk, coupons for movie rentals or other entertainment, or art supplies.

✦ Create a non-food "theme" basket, such as a basket filled with arts and crafts supplies, or a basket with (safe) play dough and an assortment of cookie cutters.

HALLOWEEN

Halloween can be an especially difficult holiday for food-allergic children, especially those that are very young. "Trick-or-Treating" (i.e., going door to door throughout the neighborhood to collect candy) is quite popular in most parts of the U.S. Many of the individually wrapped pieces of candy that are passed out on Halloween do not contain an ingredient statement, and you are likely to find that most of those that do have an ingredient statement are not safe for your child. Some possible solutions to the "what to do about Halloween" dilemma include:

✦ **Stay Home**   If this is your first child, don't take her trick-or-treating at all until she is old enough to notice that she is being left out. Convince her that it is truly special and fun to stay home and distribute candy to the kids who come to your door. (Pity those poor other children who are missing out on the excitement of opening the door and seeing all the wonderful costumes).

✦ **Distribute Safe Candy to Your Neighbors**   If your child is very young and you are on good terms with your neighbors, "secretly" go around the neighborhood in advance of Halloween night and distribute safe candy for your neighbors to give to your child when you come by. Ask them to do this in such a way that your child will not realize what's going on.

✦ **Go Trick-or-Treating**   Go trick-or-treating with your child. When you get home, sort out the safe candy from the unsafe candy (including all candies – even of familiar brands and varieties – that do not contain an ingredient statement). Remember that "snack size" candies often contain different ingredients or are produced on different machinery than the same company's "full size" offerings. Trade the unsafe candy for safe candy which you have purchased in advance, or for a non-food "prize."

✦ **Throw a Party**   On Halloween night, host a party at your home featuring fun activities and safe food. Don't go trick-or-treating at all.

PASSOVER

Most of the foods traditionally served during the Jewish holiday of Passover contain common allergens. Matzah contains wheat, cherositz contains nuts, matzah kugle often contains wheat, nuts, and eggs, and so forth... not to mention the hard-boiled eggs on the seder plate! It can be difficult enough to feed a food-allergic child during the rest of the year (especially if multiple food allergies are involved); a week of avoiding most grains and all leavened foods really compounds the challenge. My advice if your family keeps Kosher for Passover: Be creative. Make a fruit cherositz. Serve chicken and baked potatoes. Use a plastic egg on the ceremonial seder plate. And lower your nutritional standards for the week!

CONCLUDING THOUGHTS ABOUT PARENTING

Although raising a child with life-threatening food allergies can be very overwhelming, it is a wonderful feeling when you realize how many people are "on your team" helping to keep your child safe.

At the end of her son Nicholas' very successful first year in preschool, Michelle realized that twenty families had literally gone out of their way to learn about food allergies and to help keep her son safe. Although each of these other parents started out very frightened about the situation, no one wanted to do anything that could hurt Nicholas. As the year went on Michelle found out about some of the precautions that other parents were spontaneously taking, including not serving peanut butter or nut products at home on preschool mornings, keeping wet wipes in their cars so they could wipe their children's hands and face before school, cutting out food allergy-related articles for Michelle to read, and calling to ask how they could make it safe for Nicholas to come over and play at their homes.

Lastly, try to keep things in perspective. Some day you may realize that you've been so successful in managing your child's food allergies that he is completely at ease with his condition.

When her 8-year-old son Jake came to her dejectedly and said, "Mom, I feel so sorry for me," Barbara immediately felt the tears welling up inside of her. This was going to be it, she thought. Her son was going to let loose a river of tears bemoaning his food allergies and the unfairness of it all. Trying to hold back tears herself she looked at him and said, "What is it, Jake?"

"Mom," he said very sadly, "I'm the only kid I know who doesn't have board shorts!"

CHAPTER 7

SOCIALIZING

In our society most social situations revolve around food. For parents of food-allergic children, especially very young children who cannot watch out for themselves, attending a party – or even dropping by a friend's house for the afternoon – can feel like stepping into a minefield. Fortunately, with advance planning, your family can still enjoy a full and satisfying social life.

As I have mentioned elsewhere in this book, it is important to note that studies have shown that the majority of food-allergic children will not experience anaphylaxis if they merely touch an allergen, although a localized reaction (such as hives) may occur. There is a danger of a serious reaction occurring if your child actually ingests an allergen – even the minute quantity of allergen that would be consumed if he touched some allergenic food residue and then put his fingers in his mouth or touched and then consumed his otherwise "safe" food.

As you read this chapter, keep in mind that the precautions that you will need to take when socializing depend entirely on your child's age and the severity of his allergies. Older children generally require fewer precautions. For example, you need to assume that your one-year-old will put everything within reach into his mouth, whereas a 7-year-old can probably be relied upon to keep her fingers out of her mouth and to wash her hands before touching food.

As your child gets older, socializing becomes much easier. Of course, this is the case whether or not your child has food allergies!

HAVING GUESTS VISIT YOUR HOME

Now that you've turned your home into a "safe haven" for your food-allergic child, you will need to enlist the help of your guests to keep it safe.

YOUR GUESTS' BABIES

When your friends bring their babies into your home, you may need to take precautions to avoid allowing these infants to spit up on your carpets or furniture, especially if your food-allergic child tends to put her hands or fingers into her mouth. The food/formula/breast milk that your friends' babies spit up is likely to be allergenic, and will therefore "contaminate" the surfaces on which it lands. Because your goal is to make your home a safe haven for your child, be sure that your friends' babies are set down on a clean blanket or other appropriate carpet or furniture protector.

YOUR GUESTS' DIRTY HANDS

Because one of your goals should be to make your home a safe haven where you and your child do not need to worry about coming into contact with unexpected allergenic food residue, you need to take precautions to ensure that other people do not "contaminate" your home. When friends who have been eating just prior to seeing you drop by for a visit, explain the situation and ask them (and their children!!) to wash their hands upon arrival at your home – before they touch anything. I realize that no matter how politely you make this request you will still feel rude doing so, but this precaution will help you to maintain the safety of your home for your child.

> *When Donna invites friends who have young children to visit her home, she politely requests that the parents wash the child's hands and face prior to the visit, that they refrain from serving the child peanuts or nuts before the visit, and that they do not bring any food into Donna's home.*

ONLY SERVE "SAFE" FOOD

When you entertain in your home, consider only serving foods which are safe for your child. Doing so will make your child feel included (for a change!) and will eliminate the potential for allergenic food being spilled on your carpets or furniture, or contaminating your child's toys or food.

OVERNIGHT HOUSE GUESTS

If you invite friends to stay at your home overnight, be sure to explain to them all of the food-related "rules and procedures" that you follow in order to keep your home and your food supply safe for your child. It is especially important that your guests understand the precautions that they need to take to avoid contaminating your "safe" food with any allergenic food that you keep in the house.

One of my house guests once took the butter knife which had been on his plate next to his scrambled eggs and put it into our jar of strawberry jam. This "contaminated" the entire jar of jam. In hindsight I realized that I should have either spread the jam on all of the toast prior to serving it, or I should have placed a small amount of jam into a serving dish and placed that at the table. Although I always remember to spread jam on my toast before my knife touches my plate, it is not reasonable to expect my guests to think of this type of precaution – especially if, as was the case above, my allergic child is not home at the time to provide a visual reminder of his special needs.

If your house guests are bringing any pets, be sure to check the ingredients of the pets' food and treats.

Michelle's peanut-allergic son Nicholas ended up in the hospital Emergency Room on Christmas Day. They had house guests who had brought their dog. Michelle had discussed all of the pertinent precautions with her guests, and had even checked the ingredients of the dog's food. Evidently Michelle had not been specific enough. After the ER visit Michelle learned that the dog had been eating and playing with a peanut butter bone!

YOUR CHILD'S BIRTHDAY PARTIES

When planning a birthday party for your child, focus on the party activities rather than the food. Young children are thrilled with parties that include exciting activities and delicious dessert. They won't even notice if you do not serve lunch. Your local library should have some books available on themes and activities for children's parties.

HOST THE PARTY AT YOUR HOUSE

The safest place to hold your child's birthday party is in your own home. If you choose to hold the party at a different venue (such as a bowling alley, park, children's gym, or ceramics painting studio) you need to thoroughly assess the venue's safety from the food and food allergy standpoint.

ONLY SERVE "SAFE" FOOD

All the food served at the party should be completely safe for the birthday child. For this reason, it may be easiest to only serve dessert and drinks. Young children are usually too excited to eat a full meal, and are not likely to notice if you do not even serve snacks.

BAKE THE CAKE YOURSELF

If your child is allergic to peanuts, tree nuts, dairy products, eggs, or wheat, a store-bought birthday cake will not be safe for him.

———— ✹ ————

If you do bake a homemade birthday cake, you (and your child) are going to want it to look as attractive as possible. Learning the art of basic cake decorating is an investment that will pay off for many years, as you are likely to be baking your child's cakes for years to come. In fact, once you purchase the equipment and learn the tricks, basic cake decorating really is not that difficult. Call your local school district, community college district, crafts store, or cooking store to see if they offer an adult education course on cake decorating – and sign up.

———— ✹ ————

An alternative to decorating your cake with frosting is to purchase a cake decorating stencil at your local kitchen/cooking store, and use sifted powdered sugar (confectioner's sugar) to create an attractive design.

BIRTHDAY CAKE ALTERNATIVES

There are many good food allergy cookbooks on the market in which to look for a suitable birthday cake recipe. However, if your child's diet is so restrictive (or you are such a terrible baker) that a delicious homemade cake is not an option, then you need to "think outside the box." After all, there is no law that birthday parties must include birthday cake! The sky's the limit once you get past the "birthday cake paradigm." Depending on your child's allergies, consider serving one of the following:

✦ Jell-O® gelatin. Put out an array of sliced fruits and have a "decorate your own Jell-O®" party.

✦ Rice Krispie treats, possibly cut into fun shapes or made in a pan and then frosted and decorated to look like a cake.

✦ Ice cream (or "non-dairy frozen dessert"), with or without safe toppings.

✦ Multiple flavors of ice cream (or "non-dairy frozen dessert"), frozen in layers in a pan to create a cake-free "ice cream cake."

✦ Frozen fruit bars.

✦ "Safe" candy.

✦ Fresh fruit. Make a creative fruit arrangement and stick the candles in a pineapple!

✦ Any other safe treat you can think of.

**INTERNATIONAL
PERSPECTIVE**

COUNTRY	COMMENTS
Australia	In Australia, "Jell-O" is known as "jelly"
New Zealand	In New Zealand, "Jell-O" is known as "jelly," and "Rice Krispies" are called "Rice Bubbles" or "Ricies."

SOCIALIZING OUTSIDE OF YOUR HOME

Depending on the severity of your child's food allergies, there are a number of precautions which you need to take before attending a social event outside of your home. This is the case whether the "social event" in question is simply spending a morning at a friend's house, or if you've received an invitation to a child's birthday party, family get-together, dinner party, classroom holiday celebration, or a large-scale social function. In all cases you need to ask questions to determine whether or not the environment itself will be safe for your child (and if not, what can you do to make it so?) and whether or not the food will be safe for your child (and if not, can you simply bring your child's food from home?).

DON'T EXPECT TOO MUCH OF OTHERS

Even the most well-meaning friends frequently make mistakes. After all, creating a safe environment for your child is often an all-consuming task for you, and you're focused on it 24/7. It's not realistic to expect someone else to think of all the allergy implications of every detail of their party.

Angela took her highly allergic 2-year-old daughter, Ava, to the birthday party of Ava's good friend. The birthday child's parents had graciously worked with Angela in advance to create a safe party environment for Ava. The party host, a professional chef, had meticulously obtained Angela's approval on all of the ingredients for the food he was preparing. You can imagine Angela's surprise when she stepped into the living room to find a crowd of preschoolers greedily – and messily – gobbling up the platter full of highly allergenic chocolate truffles that had been purchased at the local chocolate store! "Oh my!" said the hosts as the chocolate-covered children ran off, "We didn't even think that those could be a problem!"

ALWAYS BRING YOUR MEDICINE PACK AND "SAFE" FOOD

When attending social events, always bring your child's emergency medication as well as an adequate supply of safe foods that he enjoys. Place your child's food in a small lunch box or cooler which can be set aside (away from the party food and away from the other guests) until your child is hungry.

Double-check that you have your child's medicine pack with you when you arrive at the party. If you have accidentally left it elsewhere, **leave the party and return when you have the medication.**

REACTIONS TO FOOD PARTICLES
IN OTHER PEOPLE'S HOMES

If your child is exceptionally sensitive, it is theoretically possible that she could have a reaction to the residue or airborne particles of a food that was consumed in large quantities in someone else's home just prior to her arrival. If this is the case, you should mention this when you make social plans. Call ahead before you leave your house to find out if your hosts have been consuming highly allergenic foods that day. If necessary, cancel or change your plans.

Within minutes of stepping into the home of some family friends for a holiday visit, Angela's peanut-allergic daughter, Ava, began to have a fairly severe allergic reaction. After a frightening trip to the hospital, Angela had a long chat with her hosts. She learned that throughout the day the family had been enjoying a large bowl of peanut-based trail mix. The previous evening the family had been eating peanut brittle. Ava had been given a stuffed animal when they walked in the door. Angela concluded that the likely trigger of the reaction was either the airborne peanut particles that were throughout the house from the trail mix, inhalation of peanut particles that were on the stuffed animal, or ingestion of peanut particles that were on the stuffed animal if Ava had put her fingers in her mouth after touching the toy (she was a thumb sucker at the time). Of course, Angela will never know what triggered the reaction – but this incident has made her quite leery of social outings.

REQUEST A NUT-FREE ENVIRONMENT

If your child has severe peanut or tree nut allergies, it may not be safe for her to attend a social function at which dishes of nuts will be set out for guests to enjoy. You may be particularly concerned about the dangers posed by the residue that is likely to get transferred from the other guests' hands to objects around the house – especially if there will be other children at the party. If this is a concern, then when you receive an invitation and make your initial call to the hostess, ask if it would be possible for her to refrain from setting out dishes of nuts. Make it clear that if dishes of nuts will be set out, you and your child will not be able to attend.

One time Anjali was told by a friend that she would be serving peanuts at her party. The friend just did not "get it" that this would be a severe hazard for Anjali's daughter. Finally Anjali and her husband Sam called the friend back and said that their family would not be able to attend the party. Rather than making up a "polite" excuse, they were honest about their reason for declining the invitation. The friend immediately said that she would change the menu because she wanted them to attend. Anjali and her family went to the party and had a great time!

LETTING OTHERS COOK FOR YOUR CHILD

One of the very difficult things that you will need to do as the parent of a severely food-allergic child is to figure out which of your friends and relatives you can trust to learn to safely cook for your child, and which you cannot. Although not all of your friends or relatives will be interested in trying to cook for your child, there are bound to be some who offer but who are likely to make mistakes in the process.

———— ❧ ————

As you have learned in Chapters 3, 4, and 5, purchasing and preparing food for a severely food-allergic child is not a simple matter. Before allowing a friend or relative to cook for your child, you must assess (based on your knowledge of this person) whether or not this person is willing and able to follow all of the necessary precautions. If you believe this person is both willing to learn and capable of following through, a good way to start the teaching process is to review chapters 3, 4 and 5 of this book with him or her. If you do not feel that you would be comfortable feeding your child food which was prepared by this person, thank him or her profusely for considering taking on this responsibility, and then politely decline the offer.

ASK THE HOSTESS ABOUT THE MENU

When attending a social gathering, some parents of food-allergic children prefer to bring all of their child's food from home, whereas others like to find out in advance if any of the food being served will be safe for their child.

When you receive a social invitation, contact the host/hostess to explain your child's special needs. Find out if there is anything on the menu (especially finger food) that is so highly allergenic that your child cannot safely be near it, or if there is anything on the menu (such as a packaged product) that might be safe for your child to eat. Be sure to ask about all snack foods which will be set out, in addition to foods being served at the meal itself.

If a safe packaged food will be served, ask the hostess to save the packaging for you to double-check when you arrive. Also, be sure that a fresh package is opened. Chances are high that the open package which your hostess has in her pantry is contaminated with food residue, such as from someone's hand.

IF THE HOSTESS PLANS TO COOK SOMETHING "SAFE"

Even if your friends and family are willing to attempt to prepare food for your child, you need to decide if it is worth the risk of error. Sometimes, especially for large parties where many people who do not know your child may offer to help out in the kitchen, it is easiest to simply bring your child's food from home.

> *"For us, given the severity of our children's food allergies, we now don't take any chances," says Laura, mother of two food-allergic boys. "Even at Grandma's for special occasion dinners with fancy desserts, we bring food for our sons. It keeps the big meal from turning into a bigger event with blaring sirens and four-hour hospital stays."*

If your hostess is planning to cook something which she plans to serve to your child, ask the same questions of her that you would ask of a restaurant manager or chef (see page 106).

When you arrive at the party, politely repeat all of your questions regarding the dish's ingredients and preparation. Mistakes can easily happen.

> *Many years ago a well-meaning friend prepared a special batch of cookies to be served at her son's birthday party, using a dairy-, egg-, and nut-free recipe which I had provided. Just before handing my son a cookie I asked a few polite questions – and found out that she had used real butter to grease the cookie sheet before adding the dairy-free cookie dough!*

KEEPING "SAFE" FOODS SAFE

When a dish of food is put out that is safe for your child, make sure that it will not be contaminated with allergenic foods. For example, do not place your child's safe potato chips next to a bowl full of allergenic dip, as it is possible for stray bits of dip to fall into the chips.

———————

When you bring a "safe" dish to be served at a social get-together, bring it completely covered. Place a note on top of the dish which reads, "Please keep covered and separate until (your child's name) has been served."

I once watched as whipped cream from another dessert fell onto the covered serving platter containing the dairy-free cookies which I had brought to the get-together. If the platter had not been covered, my son would not have been able to have dessert.

If your child is attending a party at which only certain menu items are safe for him to eat (such as a class party at which he can only eat the store-bought potato chips brought by another parent and the fruit salad prepared by you), arrange for your child to be served first, before the food can become contaminated by the allergenic dishes. Make sure that anyone who touches his food will do so with clean hands.

BE WARY OF INGREDIENTS OF PARTY FOODS

Never make any assumptions about the ingredients of foods being served at a party, even if you are at a family gathering where all of the chefs are familiar with your child's situation. You never know what the "secret ingredient" might be or what last-minute substitutions were made.

———————

If stuffed poultry is being served (such as for Thanksgiving or Christmas dinner), be sure to inquire about the ingredients of the stuffing. If your child is allergic to any of the stuffing ingredients, the poultry will not be safe for your child either. Also, don't forget to inquire about the ingredients of the poultry itself. For example, in the U.S. many turkeys are sold pre-injected with a broth solution that contains a variety of potentially allergenic ingredients.

———————

When at other people's homes, be especially wary of open jars of condiments, such as jam or honey. There is a good chance that these items have been cross-contaminated by something allergenic.

OFFER TO BRING A DESSERT

When you and your family are invited to a social event at someone's home, volunteer to bring a delicious "hypo-allergenic" dessert that can be shared with everyone. Most children love sweets. Your child will enjoy having the same dessert as everyone else. It's no fun to eat your own "special" dessert while everyone else raves about something which you can't have.

SHOW YOUR CHILD THE "SAFE" FOODS

When attending a party with a food-allergic child who is no longer a baby, show him exactly which foods at this party are safe for him. Explain to him that he should not touch any of the other foods. If the only safe foods are the ones which you brought from home, say so. If your child is young you will still need to keep a close eye on him, but eventually he will reach an age when you will be able to trust him not to touch any unsafe items at parties.

I started doing this with my children when they were toddlers, and by the time they were 3 or 4 they understood that the other foods were all off-limits.

REMOVE DANGEROUS FOODS

If you arrive at a party with your young food-allergic child and discover that dishes of tempting but highly allergenic foods have been placed at your child's eye level, ask the hostess if you can move these items out of sight. However, be forewarned – out of sight is not necessarily out of reach!

When my son Kevin was about two we attended a family get-together at which a dish of brightly colored allergenic candies had been placed on an end table. Upon arriving at the party, I moved the dish up high onto a book shelf. Later in the day I turned my head away for a moment only to find Kevin climbing up the side of the bookcase in an attempt to reach these candies!

TELL OTHER ADULT PARTY GUESTS
ABOUT YOUR CHILD'S FOOD ALLERGIES

When attending a party with a food-allergic child who is too young to speak for herself, explain the situation to the other adults at the party and ask them not to feed anything to your child.

At large family gatherings, Michelle waits until everyone has arrived and then calls a family meeting to remind her relatives about Nicholas' allergies. She has found that even though her family members all know of Nicholas' condition, the details tend to be forgotten. "Out of sight, out of mind" prevails.

VIGILANTLY WATCH
YOUR YOUNG FOOD-ALLERGIC CHILD

Even if you have asked the other adults at a party not to feed anything to your child, do not assume that they will follow your instructions – or that every adult present at the party heard your instructions. In a party situation, you must vigilantly watch over your young food-allergic child.

When her son Beau was 18 months old, Ann took Beau and his older sister to a family birthday party. After everyone had arrived Ann literally "stopped the party" to introduce Beau, explain the situation, and ask the other guests not to give him anything to eat. Later in the day, after the other guests had eaten, Ann let her guard down for one minute to go into the kitchen to get herself a piece of cake. Beau's grandmother immediately came running. Someone (an older woman who had arrived after Ann's speech) had shared her ice cream with Beau, and Beau was now having an allergic reaction.

If you are not available to keep a constant vigilant watch over your young child throughout a party, be sure that a designated, trusted adult has taken this responsibility. Make sure that this person knows where the emergency medication is and has been trained in the procedures to follow in case your child has an allergic reaction. If you take your young food-allergic child to a party, someone needs to stay at his side throughout the event.

Remember, you are ultimately responsible for your child's safety. Do not expect the host/hostess or other guests to assume this responsibility for you.

THANK THE HOSTS

After attending a social event, be sure to thank the hosts for their efforts to accommodate your child's special needs.

OTHER CHILDREN'S BIRTHDAY PARTIES

Young children's birthday parties pose special challenges above and beyond those found at other social gatherings. From the food allergy perspective you must contend with young and excited children eating messy (and probably allergenic) food; allergenic treats served as snacks, used as game prizes, and given out in take-home bags; and a myriad of supervision issues. In addition to all of the steps that you would normally take to make your child's attendance at a party or other social event as safe as possible (see above), there are a number of additional things that you should do.

KEEP A SUPPLY OF SAFE TREATS AVAILABLE

Keep a supply of safe cupcakes or other appropriate treats in your freezer so that you will always have dessert on hand for your child to take to a birthday party.

PLAN TO STAY AT THE PARTY WITH YOUR CHILD

Until your child is old enough to handle both expected and unexpected situations (possibly around the age of 10 or 11 or even older), you must stay with him at parties, including birthday parties. As long as you're staying, offer to pitch in and be helpful. Pour drinks, clear the dirty dishes, set up a game – but always keep your child within view. Make yourself a welcome addition, so that your omnipresence at parties (which will continue for years past the point at which other parents are just dropping their children off and returning when the party is over) will always be appreciated.

CALL THE HOSTESS TO DISCUSS YOUR CHILD'S SPECIAL NEEDS

If your child's allergies are extremely severe, you will need to call the hostess prior to accepting the invitation, to determine the relative safety of the party environment. Depending on the foods being served and the activities planned (and the severity of your child's allergies), the party may not be safe for your child to attend. Try to become comfortable with calling the hostess in advance, explaining your child's situation, and making polite but detailed inquiries of the party plans – including food, activities, and entertainment.

———— ❧ ————

It is a good idea to make one fairly long call to the hostess when the invitation is received to ask all of your questions, and then to make a second much shorter call to the hostess the day before the event (after the party food has been purchased).

———— ❧ ————

During the first call you should explain your situation, emphasize that you will be staying at the party to watch over your child, and ask about all of the details of the party plan. Make it clear that you are just trying to determine if it is safe for your child to attend the party. Be extremely polite and as undemanding as possible. If the hostess expresses an interest and willingness to create a reasonably safe party environment for your child, be sure to express your gratitude. Depending on the age of your child and the other party guests you might ask:

✦ What food will be served (including meal, snacks, desserts, and beverages) at the party?

✦ If allergenic foods will be served, would the hostess be willing to only serve these items in a controlled situation at a table (i.e., to not allow children to wander around the party eating these foods)?

✦ If allergenic foods will be served, would the hostess be willing to work with you to ensure that the children go straight from the table to a sink to wash up? Note that young children require adult supervision in this washing up, to ensure that the children do not merely wipe their dirty hands and faces off on a towel.

✦ If you have a severely milk-allergic child under the age of 5 who has been invited to a party of other young children, ask the hostess if she can avoid serving milk at the party. At this age, the chances that one (or all!) of the children will spill their milk is very high, and this spilled milk can pose a large danger to your child.

✦ Do any of the planned activities (including art projects and games) involve food?

✦ If any of the planned activities would be particularly dangerous for your child (such as an egg toss game, a "make your own peanut butter sandwich" activity, or a pie eating contest), could the plans be changed?

✦ Will there be any outside entertainment (such as clowns or magicians)? If so, would it be possible for you to call this entertainer to inquire about food used during his presentation?

✦ In general, is the other parent willing to work with you to create a reasonably safe situation for your child?

Based on the hostess' answers to these questions, you must determine if the party will be reasonably safe for your child.

During your second call to the hostess (the day before the event), you should:

✦ Emphasize that since you'll be there throughout the party she can count on your help in supervising all of the children.

✦ Ask the hostess to save the packaging for any foods being served that might be safe for your child (such as potato chips and punch), so that you can double-check the ingredients when you arrive.

✦ Re-inquire about anything that would pose a particularly major safety hazard for your child (such as bowls of nuts on the table or craft projects that involve food).

✦ Ask the hostess not to put allergenic candy in your child's take-home "goody" bag.

CALL ANY HIRED ENTERTAINERS

If entertainers (such as clowns, magicians, and so forth) are being hired for the event, you might want to obtain the entertainer's telephone number and contact him well in advance of the party. Explain your child's situation to the entertainer, and find out if he uses food in any way as part of his act. For example, many entertainers distribute candy to reward children for participation, magicians may make a food item "magically" appear (and touch the volunteer's skin in the process), and science teachers may lead the children in a food-based experiment. Some entertainers regularly throw peanuts or candies at the crowd! The entertainer's answers will help you determine if the party will be a safe situation for your child.

BRING FOOD FOR YOUR CHILD

Find out what food will be served at the party and try to bring a similar (but safe) alternative for your child.

SEAT YOUR CHILD AT THE EDGE OF THE TABLE

If all of the children are to be seated for a meal and/or dessert, arrange to have your child seated at the edge of the table, next to a child who is known to be a relatively neat eater. This will cut down on the risk that your child will be touched by a child whose hands are covered with allergenic food or that your child's food will be contaminated by food that has been splattered about by a messy party guest. This type of thing is particularly a problem when the guests are 1 to 6 years old.

WATCH OUT FOR PIÑATAS

Candy-filled piñatas are especially popular in some areas. The children take turns hitting at the piñata with a stick or baseball bat until it breaks open, causing the candy to fall onto the ground. All of the children then rush forward to scoop up as much candy as they can. If the piñata is filled with allergenic treats, you will need to decide if it is safe for your child to even touch this candy (so that you could later trade that candy for safe candy).

When my son was in preschool we attended a birthday party that was held outside on a particularly hot August day. The piñata, which had been filled and hung up earlier in the day, was saved as the last activity of the day (after the very popular "run through the sprinklers" activity). The birthday child's parents obviously had not thought things through, as they had filled the piñata with snack-sized chocolate treats. When the piñata broke open a mass of melted, sticky (and highly allergenic) chocolate goo fell to the patio. We had to leave immediately, as it was no longer safe for us to be there.

CHILDREN'S PLAY DATES

When your child is invited to another child's home to play, there are three main questions which need to be answered:

1. Who will be responsible for your child's safety (i.e., will you be staying or will the other parent be responsible)?

2. Will it be a safe environment for your child?

3. What (if anything) will your child – and the other child – be eating?

TALK TO THE OTHER PARENT

When your child first receives an invitation to another child's house, you need to have a frank discussion with the other parent about your child's food allergies and their seriousness. Explain that your child has severe, potentially fatal food allergies, and that if you are not going to be staying for this play date then you will need to spend 15 minutes with the other parent going over the emergency procedures which need to be followed in case of a reaction. Ask the other parent if he/she is comfortable assuming this responsibility. If the answer is "no," offer to stay or to have the children get together at your house. If the answer is "yes," see pages 29-30 regarding training others in your child's emergency procedures.

———✦———

A particularly difficult topic to bring up when your child is invited to another child's home to play is the issue of household cleanliness. If the other family routinely allows family members to eat throughout the house – especially if toddlers or preschoolers are permitted to walk around the home munching on whatever your child is allergic to – the environment may not be safe for your child. Asking about this while avoiding insulting the other parent can be quite tricky. After telling the other parent about the seriousness of your child's allergies you may want to say something like, "Suzie's allergies are so severe that we even need to be concerned about small bits of food residue that she might touch. I know that most families do not confine food to the kitchen table, and they may eat sandwiches, snacks, and other finger foods while working or playing throughout the house. What are the chances, for example, that there might be peanut butter or cheese residue on Jennifer's toys or on your furniture? This is the type of thing which we would need to be concerned about during Suzie's visit."

———— ❧ ————

If your severely peanut-allergic child has been invited to play at a friend's home, be sure to explain to the other parent that it would not be safe for their family members to consume peanut butter or other peanut products while your child is there.

———— ❧ ————

If you will not be staying for the play date, make sure that the other parent knows how to reach you in case there is any type of problem or question.

BRING THE MEDICINE PACK
If you will be dropping your child off, be sure that you leave your child's medicine pack with the (fully trained) other parent – and don't forget to take it back with you when you pick your child up at the end of the play date.

SEND "SAFE" FOOD
Unless you know the other parent very well and truly trust her to prepare food for your child, always insist on sending all the snacks and meals which your child will consume on a play date at someone else's home. It is often a good idea to send enough snack food for the other child and the other child's siblings as well.

WASH HANDS
Ask the other parent to ensure that all family members (especially your child's playmate) wash their hands with soap if they have eaten something to which your child is allergic prior to your child's arrival or during your child's visit.

———— ❧ ————

Politely remind the other parent that she needs to wash her hands with soap before touching your child's food, including any "safe" food which you brought for your child. You do not want her to contaminate the food when she serves it.

CLEAN HIGH CHAIRS AND WASHCLOTHS

If your food-allergic toddler is going to eat while at a friend's home, be sure to thoroughly wipe down the other child's high chair before allowing your child to sit in it. In addition, be sure that after eating, your child's face and hands are wiped off with a clean washcloth – not the cloth which was used on the other child.

When my son was a toddler, another mother generously offered to watch him for 3 or 4 hours. She was quite familiar with his allergies, we had gone over all of the emergency procedures, and I had sent safe food for him to eat. On a previous visit I had seen that she kept a very clean house, and she told me that her son ate all his meals and snacks in his highchair. It was as safe a situation as possible. When Jason got hungry my friend set him in her son's highchair to eat; when he was done she unthinkingly grabbed the washcloth which was on the counter and wiped his face. His face immediately turned bright red. She quickly got him out of the highchair to assess the situation, and saw that the backs of his legs were covered in hives. Luckily the antihistamine which she gave him stopped the reaction within minutes, but she did have a good scare. Upon reflection we realized that (a) the high chair seat was not clean, and (b) the washcloth was full of milk residue from her son's breakfast.

OVERNIGHT VISITS

By the time your child is school age, she is likely to want to have overnight visits with her close friends. If your child is invited to spend the night at a friend's home, you should follow all of the precautions that you would for any other play date and/or party. You will probably find it easiest (and least stressful for both you and the host family) to send all of the food that your child will be consuming.

————◆————

For slumber parties, you need to ensure that highly allergenic foods will not be served at the party at all. This will greatly lower the risk factor for your child. There is a good chance that the host parents will not even be in the room when snacks are served. For example, it is not safe for your highly milk-allergic child to be sitting on the sofa (or lounging on a pile of sleeping bags) with a group of children who are all eating popcorn with melted butter. The butter residue will get on everything in the room, creating an unsafe situation for your child.

EMOTIONAL ISSUES

All of the precautions that you need to take and all of the questions that you need to ask before taking your child to another person's home are bound to start to make you feel like a social "wet blanket." My best advice (which, unfortunately, is fairly harsh) is to get over it. Your child has special needs. You cannot force your family into the same mode of living that other families (who are not dealing with the challenge of life-threatening food allergies) enjoy. What you can do is to create a new life for you and your family that is both joyous and as "normal" as possible. Accept the fact that you can no longer take a carefree approach to life and just do your best to maintain a positive and upbeat attitude.

As parents we may feel sad that we are always sending our children to social events with a lunchbox of food. We feel they are missing out on a wonderful aspect of life. Food is very much a part of our culture, and social events are associated with an opportunity to eat "special" food. Try to keep in mind, though, that if your child has spent his entire life not eating the food at parties, he might not feel left out at all. Given a choice, he may even prefer the favorites that you have packed for him to the "strange" food that everyone else is eating.

When my son was young, I always brought a "special" cupcake for him to eat at birthday parties. Inevitably, one or two of the other children would announce that Jason's cupcake looked more appealing than the birthday cake which was being served, and would ask for one just like his!

In fact, sometimes it can be quite an advantage to bring your own food to a party. When Jason was in seventh grade he was chosen as a "Student of the Trimester," and was invited to sit with his teacher at the "Student of the Trimester Luncheon." The event was catered by the school cafeteria, and the food was evidently inedible....Jason's teacher took one bite and stated that the tacos "tasted like dog meat." Everyone was jealous as they watched Jason enjoy the delicious lunch that he had brought from home!

CHAPTER 8

OUTINGS

———◆———

Like all families, your family can enjoy visits to parks, zoos, movie theatres, museums, amusement parks, and so forth. Most food-allergic children are able to safely enjoy most outings of this sort with only a relatively small amount of "extra preparation hassle" on your part.

———◆———

Unfortunately, if your child is one of the minority of food-allergic children who react to airborne particles of allergens, going just about anywhere can become quite complicated. In this case you will need to give a lot of advance thought (and possible research) to exactly what you are likely to encounter at your destination... and then make an educated guess as to whether or not the situation will be safe for your child.

> *Angela's daughter, Ava, felt ill after walking by a large open display of free samples of flavored nuts that was set up in the walkway area of their local shopping mall. Gail's daughter, Sara, reacted to airborne particles from the Rotisserie Grilled Chicken that was being cooked in the deli area of their supermarket.*

GENERAL THINGS TO KEEP IN MIND

BRING THE MEDICINE PACK

Don't forget that whenever you take your child anywhere, her emergency medication pack needs to be close at hand. A convenient way to carry your child's medicine pack on outings is in a fanny pack.

BRING FOOD

Whenever you go somewhere with your child you should bring along something safe for her to eat, in case she gets hungry. Unlike other parents, you cannot count on just "picking up something" at your destination.

Julie likes to keep a bag that is always packed with a selection of shelf-stable snacks that are safe for her 2-year-old daughter, Autumn. When they're ready to go somewhere, Julie just grabs this bag as one of the things to bring along. When they return home Julie refills it so it will be ready for next time.

BE FLEXIBLE

Be prepared to be flexible – or even to cancel your plans – if a situation turns out to be unsafe for your child. For example, a restaurant that was popular when I was in college had peanut shells covering the floor as part of the décor. If you and your peanut-allergic child should unexpectedly encounter a similar situation, be prepared to turn around and leave at once.

CONSIDER SPECIAL ALLERGY BUTTONS AND CLOTHING

When your child is young, you may wish to have her wear a special "allergy button" or specialized "allergy clothing" when you go on outings. Although you will be watching her at all times throughout the outing, this is just an extra precaution that you can take to alert others to her condition.

———◈———

Many crafts stores sell blank 3-inch diameter buttons which you can personalize and then pin onto your toddler or preschooler's clothing whenever you leave the house. Possible wording for your child's brightly colored button includes "Severely Allergic to Peanuts and Eggs" or "I Have Food Allergies - Please Do Not Feed Me." See Appendix H for sample artwork. Some internet-based vendors sell buttons or stickers with similar messages.

———◈———

There are a variety of internet-based sources for children's T-shirts, sweatshirts, and other articles of clothing which contain a food allergy message (such as "nut free zone") as part of the design. Some of these are listed on the links page of my website, www.FoodAllergyBooks.com.

PURCHASE A BACKPACK

Once your family no longer needs to bring a stroller on outings, you should invest in a comfortable backpack or knapsack in which you can carry your child's food on trips to amusement parks and other all-day outings.

I own a wonderful two-part knapsack: The bottom is a small insulated soft-sided cooler, and the top is a large section for non-refrigerated items (such as crackers and jackets).

SPECIFIC ADVICE FOR
SPECIFIC DESTINATIONS

PARKS AND PLAYGROUNDS

When you first arrive at a playground, take a quick look at the playground equipment to see if there is any obvious, visible food residue on it. If so, use a wet wipe to clean it up.

———————

Watch out for well-meaning mothers (or other children) who may offer a snack to your child.

———————

As in all away-from-home situations, always stay within an arm's reach distance of your food-allergic toddler while you are at a park. You never know what she might pick up off the ground and attempt to put into her mouth.

———————

Carry your child's medicine pack with you while you are at the park. You should not set it down somewhere unattended where it could pose a danger to some other curious child.

PLAY AREAS AT FAST FOOD RESTAURANTS

Many fast food restaurants have special children's play areas with climbing tubes, tunnels, ball pits, and more. Because of its location within a restaurant, this playground equipment is often covered with a great deal of food residue. If your child is very sensitive to any of the ingredients of the foods commonly served at the restaurant (or if she tends to suck her thumb or put her fingers in her mouth), it may not be safe for her to play on this equipment at all.

MOVIE THEATRES

If you are concerned that your child might react to the food residue that is on the seat at the movie theatre, it is relatively simple to create a "safe" movie theatre experience for your child:

❏ Bring a wet washcloth or wet wipe (or get a wet paper towel from the restroom) and wipe down your child's seat and armrests.

❏ If necessary, you can also bring a beach towel to place on your child's seat, and then have her sit on this towel.

❏ Seat your child either in the middle of your group or on an aisle seat next to you; do not permit anyone in your group to eat anything allergenic.

AMUSEMENT PARKS

In recent years many amusement parks have become more aware of severe food allergies, and many will attempt to accommodate the needs of your food-allergic child. Call the park at least one week prior to your trip and talk to the Head Chef or the Food Service Manager. Find out what, if anything, the park serves or sells that would be safe for your child. There may be some prepackaged food (such as potato chips or frozen fruit bars) available that are safe, or you may be able to arrange for the chef to cook something special for your child. If the park will be cooking food for your child, treat this situation the same as you would treat any restaurant visit (see Chapter 9).

———— ✦ ————

If you do not want to go through the hassle of making advance arrangements for your child's food needs, you can simply bring all of your child's food with you. Be aware, however, that some amusement parks have official policies which forbid you from bringing in any outside food. Most will relax this policy if you explain your child's special situation. However, if you do run into problems with this in the U.S., you can explain to the park personnel that your child is covered by the A.D.A. (Americans with Disabilities Act), and that this law requires the park to accommodate your child. Rather than asking the amusement park to prepare food for your child – which the park would have to guarantee is 100% free of any trace of allergen – you are merely asking for the extremely reasonable accommodation of allowing you to bring in food for your child. Point out that you will be purchasing food for the other members of your group. If you put it this way, the park personnel will probably not give you any further argument.

———— ✦ ————

While at the amusement park, avoid purchasing any messy allergenic foods for others in your group.

MUSEUMS AND AQUARIUMS

Many children's museums, aquariums, and other water-themed places have "touch tanks" where children can touch star fish, anemones, crabs, and other aquatic creatures. If your child is extremely sensitive to fish or shell fish, she may have a reaction simply from sticking her hand in the touch tank. In this case, simply enjoy the other exhibits and steer clear of the touch tanks.

———— ✦ ————

Many science museums and children's museums have interactive exhibits (such as paleontology exhibits at which children can pretend to dig for dinosaur bones) in which ground walnut shells are used in place of sand or dirt. If your child is allergic to nuts, call the museum in advance of your visit to find out if there are any exhibits which you will need to avoid. If your child is extremely sensitive to nuts, you will need to evaluate whether the nut residue that may be on all of the other interactive exhibits at this museum (due to the residue on the other visitors' hands) or that may be in the air will pose a risk to your child.

BALL GAMES

If your child is allergic to peanuts, creating a safe environment at a ball game (where bags of peanuts are extremely popular snack items) can be a challenge. You may find yourself in a situation where the ground around you is literally covered with peanut shells.

 INTERNATIONAL PERSPECTIVE

COUNTRY	COMMENTS
United Kingdom	Football (soccer) matches are most commonly attended in the U.K. Peanuts do not appear to be a major hazard at such events.

If your child reacts to airborne peanut particles, he will not be safe in a ball game environment unless you can arrange for an entire peanut-free section. Some parents have succeeded in making this arrangement, and some have not. Call the management of the ball park very far in advance of the game which you would like to attend. You are more likely to succeed if you have a large group of people who are interested in purchasing tickets to sit in this peanut-free zone with you, and if you are willing to attend a less popular game (don't expect such concessions from the ball team for the play-off games!). Small minor-league teams are also more likely to be able to cooperate with this request than are major-league teams.

If you are taking your peanut-allergic child to a ball game at which you will not be sitting in a peanut-free zone, you can minimize the risk by doing the following:

❑ Have your child wear long pants and long sleeves, so most of her skin will not come in contact with allergens.

❑ Bring a wet washcloth or wet wipe and use it to wipe down your child's seat and armrests.

❑ Explain your situation to the strangers who are sitting next to and behind you. Politely ask them not to throw any peanuts or peanut shells, and ask them to please keep their peanut shells as far away from your child as possible. Perhaps you can even offer them a plastic grocery bag (which you brought for this reason) in which to place their peanut shells.

❑ Seat your child in the middle of your group so that he will not be seated next to anyone who is eating peanuts.

❑ Do not set any of your possessions (such as backpacks, jackets, etc.) under your seat, where they are likely to come into contact with peanut shells, peanut particles and peanut dust. Keep everything on your lap.

❑ As with most outings in your life now, you will most likely need to bring your child's food from home. If you would like to purchase food for your child at the ball game, call the Food Service Manager in advance to determine the safety of the available food. Treat this situation the same as you would treat any restaurant visit (see Chapter 9).

CHAPTER 9

RESTAURANTS

Taking a child who has severe food allergies to a restaurant can be quite problematic, and many parents choose to simply avoid it altogether. Many restaurants cannot readily tell you the ingredients of their food; the risks of "safe" food becoming contaminated with allergens in the restaurant kitchen are enormous; and, especially if your child has multiple allergies, there may not be anything on the menu which does not contain something to which your child is allergic. If your child is very young you can simply bring her food from home. With an older child, however, this option is not always comfortable or appropriate (or permitted by the restaurant itself).

If you do choose to try to take your child to a restaurant, you will need to take many precautions and be extra-vigilant.

DON'T ASSUME A RESTAURANT WILL BE ABLE TO ACCOMMODATE YOU

A restaurant may be unable, or unwilling, to accommodate your child's special needs.

I recently took my peanut-, tree nut-, and egg-allergic son to a restaurant that is known for its very broad menu. The restaurant manager and I discussed Jason's special needs and determined that he could not eat anything that came from their deep fryer (some of their fried menu items were coated in an egg batter), anything from their grill (one popular item had a Thai peanut sauce, so the manager felt the cross-contamination risk for anything from their grill was high), anything from their salad bar (we always avoid salad bars, and this one had eggs, peanuts, and dishes containing mayonnaise), or anything from their pizza oven (because they still accommodated requests for the pizza with Thai chicken and peanut sauce that was no longer on their menu). Out of a multi-page menu the only safe choice was the ribs (which were cooked in the oven), with freshly washed strawberries and a plain baked potato. Even with this choice, the restaurant manager insisted on personally watching over Jason's order, to ensure that his food didn't touch anything during its journey from the oven to his plate.

AVOID BUSY TIMES AND HOLIDAYS

Avoid going to restaurants during their busiest hours or on their busiest days, when the staff will not have time to properly deal with your child's special food handling needs. If you must take your food-allergic child to a restaurant on a busy holiday, obtain permission from the restaurant manager to bring his food from home.

HIGH-RISK SITUATIONS
FOR THE FOOD ALLERGIC

Depending on what your child is allergic to, there are many situations which should be avoided altogether.

✦ **Buffets and Salad Bars**   People with severe food allergies should avoid buffets and self-service salad bars, because of the high risk of cross-contamination. Customers often contaminate items by using the same serving utensil for several dishes. In addition, food pieces may fall from one item into another while customers are serving themselves.

✦ **Bakeries**   People with severe nut allergies are generally advised to avoid all food from bakeries, because of the very high risk of cross-contamination. Many bakery items contain nuts (either whole, ground, chopped, or in paste form). Most bakeries do not wash out their bowls, baking sheets, and utensils in between batches; items are merely wiped off before being used to make a different item, and are then washed thoroughly by the end of the day. Do not serve fresh bakery goods to your tree nut- or peanut-allergic child.

Most baked goods also contain milk, egg, and wheat ingredients.

✦ **Asian Restaurants**   If your child has peanut or tree nut allergies, it is best for her to avoid food from Asian restaurants because of the very high risk of cross-contamination. Many popular Asian dishes contain nuts, and many Asian restaurants use peanut oil in their cooking. Most Asian restaurants do not wash out their woks in between batches of different dishes. In addition, they may use the same utensils to simultaneously cook several different dishes.

✦ **African, Thai, and Indian Restaurants**
If your child has peanut or tree nut allergies, she should also avoid food from African, Thai, and many Indian restaurants.

✦ **Seafood Restaurants**
People with fish or shellfish allergies should avoid all food from seafood restaurants because of the high risk of cross-contamination, and because of the high concentration of air-borne fish protein particles found within the restaurant.

✦ **Ice Cream Shops**
"Hard serve" ice cream from ice cream shops (i.e., the type that is dished up with a scoop) is not safe for most food-allergic children because of the high risk of cross-contamination. Most shops use the same scoop for all of their flavors, and merely rinse the scoop off (in a bowl of residue-filled water) in between flavors. In addition to the nut flavors (such as Peanut Butter Chocolate and Rocky Road), some popular ice cream flavors contain egg (French Vanilla), wheat (Chocolate Brownie Fudge) and other allergenic ingredients. Even if the shop shows you a complete ingredient statement and then agrees to open a fresh container of ice cream and use a freshly washed scoop for your child, you still need to determine if the ice cream itself may have come into contact with allergens during the production process (see Appendix J for a sample script to use when contacting food manufacturers).

In addition, toppings from ice cream shops are also very risky for those with food allergies, as the different toppings are often served using the same utensil, and bits of one topping frequently fall into the container which holds another topping. There can be nuts in the sprinkles, sprinkles in the cookie bits, and so forth.

ASSESS YOUR CHILD'S SITUATION

One of the biggest problems with food prepared in a restaurant setting is the cross-contamination between different dishes that takes place in the restaurant kitchen. Before contacting any restaurants, you need to know just how severe your child's allergies are. What is the likelihood that your child will react to this type of cross-contamination? If the chances are low, many of the issues raised in this chapter will not apply to your situation.

When Barbara's son Jake was young he was allergic to dairy products, yet he could safely eat a hamburger patty that had been cooked on the same grill (and probably touched with the same spatula) as the cheeseburgers. My own son, however, would have reacted to anything which had been cooked on that same grill, touched by that spatula, or touched by someone who had allergenic residue on their fingers.

SPEAK TO THE RESTAURANT MANAGER BEFORE YOUR VISIT

Before visiting a restaurant, call first and talk to the manager or the chef. Explain your child's situation. Emphasize that the problem can be fatal. Ask what menu items, if any, may be safe. Discuss the risk of cross-contamination between the theoretically "safe" menu items and the unsafe menu items. Only take your child to the restaurant if you feel confident that his needs will be met. Then, once you arrive at the restaurant, speak to the manager and/or chef and review all of the ingredients and procedures again. Do not hold this discussion with the wait person, as the wait staff is probably not qualified to answer your questions. Some of the questions/issues to discuss with the manager or chef are:

❏ Does the dish contain any [allergen] ingredients?

❏ If your child is allergic to peanuts, are peanuts or peanut butter used as a "secret ingredient" in any of their dishes or sauces?

❏ Does the person to whom you are speaking truly understand exactly what your child cannot eat? For instance, if you say he is allergic to "milk," does the chef realize that this broad category includes butter, cheese, sour cream, etc. – plus casein, whey, lactose, and so forth?

❏ Is anything brushed on the food during the cooking process? For example, many restaurants brush butter on steaks and rub oil on baked potatoes.

❏ Is the food marinated? If so, exactly what is in the marinade?

❏ Is there any sort of coating on the food? For example, I have seen French fries that contained milk, wheat, and even beef ingredients.

❏ If the restaurant receives the food partially prepared from a central commissary and simply cooks it in their kitchen, do they know the exact ingredients of each dish? (All too often, the answer is "no").

❏ What is in or on the vegetables? Do you add butter or oil? What seasonings are used? Is there any sauce?

❏ What other foods might the dish come into contact with during the preparation process? Do these foods contain any allergens?

❏ What else is cooked on the grill? Do these foods contain any allergens?

❏ If ordering anything (such as French fries) that is deep-fried: What kind of oil is used? What else is fried in the same pot of oil? Do these foods contain any allergens? Note that French fries, egg batter-coated onion rings, egg-and wheat-coated fish sticks and cheese sticks are often all fried in the same vat of oil – in these cases making all of these items unsafe for a person who is allergic to just one of these items.

❏ Is it possible for the restaurant to clean the grill, pan, spatula, knife, etc., and cook your child's food "special" – and completely separate from everything else – with one person assigned to watching over it to safeguard it from cross-contamination?

BRING THE MEDICINE PACK

When you first arrive at a restaurant, check to be sure that you have your child's emergency medicine pack with you. **If you have accidentally left it elsewhere, leave the restaurant and return when you have the medication.**

SPEAK TO THE MANAGER AGAIN BEFORE YOU ORDER

Review the ingredients and preparation of all items which you will be ordering for your food-allergic child.

In addition to speaking to the manager or chef to ask all of the pertinent questions, you may also want to give the restaurant staff a small card that briefly explains your child's food allergies (see Appendix E for a sample).

ALWAYS INQUIRE ABOUT INGREDIENTS

Even if a restaurant has posted the ingredients of a menu item (such as at juice and smoothy bars), do not assume that this is a complete listing. You still need to talk to the manager or chef.

In March 2002, after my son outgrew his dairy allergy, I called a nationwide ice cream chain to inquire about the safety of their products. I knew that they now showed an ingredient list for each item at the store, and I was calling to inquire about cross-contamination at the manufacturing plant. My thought was that perhaps the store could open up a fresh container of ice cream and scoop it up for Jason using a freshly washed scooper. I was shocked when I was told that the "ingredient list" at the store was just the "top ten ingredients" for each item – not a complete listing. Plus, of course, all of their products were produced on shared equipment with their peanut and tree nut flavors.

ORDER PLAIN, SIMPLE FOODS

When dining in a restaurant, it is usually safest to order plain, simple foods for your food-allergic child. Avoid sauces, gravies, fillings, and so forth unless you are completely sure of their ingredients.

To liven up plain salads and baked potatoes at restaurants, Marlee likes to make a dressing out of oil, balsamic vinegar, salt and pepper – ingredients which most restaurants can easily provide. She is always careful to wipe off the top of the oil and vinegar containers before using them.

AVOID MIX-UPS AND MISTAKES

When your child's food arrives, examine it for any obvious problems. If it contains visible allergens, call the manager over to discuss the problem. Insist that this plate of "contaminated" food is left at your table while a fresh dish is prepared. This ensures that the restaurant staff will not merely remove the offending items from the plate and bring the "contaminated" food back to your child.

———————

When the wait person serves your child's beverage, verbally verify what is being served. If the beverage is "hiding" in a lidded plastic cup, remove the lid and look at it to visually verify that it is the beverage which your child ordered. Mistakes do happen.

A confused waiter accidentally served Leslie's severely dairy-allergic son milk instead of a soft drink. Unfortunately, this mistake was not discovered until Jake took his first sip. This problem is not that uncommon. Barbara reports that the same thing happened to her son.

WHEN IN DOUBT, SPIT IT OUT

I mentioned this in the parenting section, but it bears repeating here. Teach your child that if he ever takes a bite or a sip of something that he suspects he is allergic to, or that just doesn't seem "right," he should immediately spit it out. This is not the time to be concerned about good manners. He should not wait until he can politely run to the restroom to spit out the offending mouthful. Regardless of the social implications, your child should spit first (perhaps into a napkin) and explain later. Remember, when in doubt, spit it out!

BRINGING FOOD FROM HOME

If you want to bring safe food from home for your child to eat at a restaurant, call ahead to obtain permission from the manager to do so. Not all restaurants permit "outside food" to be brought in.

———— ✺ ————

If you do bring food, bring something that your child will be happy to eat when served cold. Although you can ask the restaurant staff to heat your child's home-prepared meal for you, by letting the food out of your sight you risk having your child's meal (or the container in which it is stored) contaminated in the restaurant's kitchen.

DEALING WITH CONTACT SENSITIVITY ISSUES

If your child is extremely contact sensitive to food residues, it can be difficult to even bring her in to a restaurant.

> *When Gail brings her daughter Sara to a restaurant, she brings along peel-off disposable placemats. She uses three at Sara's place at the table: one on top of the table, one on the underside of the table, and one around the outer edge. This ensures that Sara only touches a completely clean surface.*

IF YOU FIND AN ACCOMMODATING RESTAURANT, STICK WITH IT!

Many times parents of children with severe food allergies find one or two local restaurants at which they have gotten to know the manager/owner/ chef, and he or she is willing to cook something "special" for their child. If you should be fortunate enough to find a similar situation, tip them generously, thank them profusely, patronize them frequently, and recommend them to your friends!

> *Julie has found a local outlet of a national chain of home-style Italian restaurants at which the chef will cook a separate pot of plain pasta for her daughter Autumn. They then supplement these noodles with the "special" food that they bring from home.*

Avo, the owner of a lovely Greek restaurant, has been cooking for Jason for all of our family's special occasions for many years. In fact, he even catered the luncheon reception for Jason's Bar Mitzvah, preparing a delicious egg- and nut-free meal for my 95 guests!

CHAPTER 10

TRAVEL

Just like so many other things in your life now, traveling with food allergies is more difficult than traveling without food allergies. You will need to determine how you will feed and create a safe environment for your child while you are on vacation.

Be flexible and relax your usual nutritional standards during your vacation. Don't worry about every meal being well-balanced. Just focus on ensuring that every meal is safe.

THINGS TO PACK WHEN YOU TRAVEL

BRING A LETTER FROM YOUR DOCTOR

It is a good idea when traveling to carry a signed letter from your doctor indicating the severity of your child's condition and the recommended emergency (and hospital emergency room) treatment. For air travel you will also need a doctor's note authorizing you to bring your EpiPens® on board the plane. Contact your doctor prior to your trip to obtain these documents. See Appendix D for sample letters. In addition, you should bring extra copies of your child's medication prescriptions.

BRING EXTRA MEDICINE PACKS

Always bring at least one extra complete medicine pack when you travel. Keep them in separate bags in case something is lost or stolen. If you don't have an extra set of medication at home, the medicine pack that is normally stored at school could be used.

BRING YOUR OWN INFANT OR CHILD SAFETY SEAT

If your child requires one, bring your own infant or child safety seat. A seat that you can rent from the airline or from a car rental service is likely to be covered in food residue. Remember, also, that in the United States laws regarding child safety seat requirements vary from state to state.

BRING YOUR OWN TOILETRIES

Bring your own "safe" soap, shampoo, lotion, and toothpaste. The products provided in hotel rooms rarely have ingredient listings and may not be safe for your child.

TRAVELING WITH OTHERS

If you are traveling with others, make sure that all of your travel companions are familiar with your child's food allergies, and are familiar with the steps that everyone in your group needs to take to keep your child safe. If appropriate, review your child's emergency care plans with the other adults in your group.

TRAVELING TO A RURAL OR FOREIGN AREA

When traveling to a rural or foreign area, call ahead to find out what telephone number to dial to call the rescue squad, where the nearest major medical center is, how the health system works, and whether the rescue squad routinely carries epinephrine. Always carry adequate insurance and cash to cover an emergency.

———————

When traveling to another country, do not make the mistake of assuming that familiar foods are identical to those available at home. For example, some foods available in the U.S. are also available in Canada – but licensed to and made by a different manufacturer (on different equipment and possibly with different ingredients). Even within the United States, products available nationwide may not all be made in the same facility.

———————

If you plan to travel outside of your country, you may wish to join the International Association for Medical Assistance to Travelers (IAMAT). This non-profit organization maintains a network of physicians who speak English and have had medical training in North America or Europe. IAMAT aims to make competent medical care available to travelers anywhere in the world. Membership is free, although donations are appreciated. Membership includes a directory of IAMAT physicians and passport-size clinical record for your doctor to complete prior to your trip. For more information, visit IAMAT's website at www.iamat.org.

BRING FOOD

Even if you have confirmed that you will be able to eat at restaurants or other people's homes once you reach your destination, you should always travel with a variety of safe ready-to-eat snacks and enough food for your child to eat for one or two meals in case there is a change in plans.

———————◦✦◦———————

Depending on your child's allergies, ideas for what to bring include:

✦ Single serving containers of applesauce or canned fruit

✦ Small boxes of raisins

✦ Snack-size bags of potato chips or pretzels

✦ Fresh fruit

✦ Crackers

✦ Cookies

✦ Small cans of tuna or chicken

✦ Small pull-top cans of vegetables or fruit

✦ Small boxes of cold cereal with shelf-stable boxes of milk (or soy milk or rice milk). Although they can be hard to find, some brands of soy milk are available in single-serving boxes, similar in size and shape to a juice box.

✦ Jars of baby food (don't overlook this option, even for an older child)

✦ Any other item which does not require refrigeration.

———————◦✦◦———————

If you are traveling with a cooler, your options will expand. For car trips, it is possible to purchase a small cooler which plugs into your car's electrical power outlet. This cooler will act as a "traveling refrigerator" in which you can bring safe food for your child. However, the plug may not also work with a regular electrical socket. If this is the case, bring along large zipper-type plastic bags which you can fill with ice at your hotel, to keep the food cold when you're not on the road.

DINING OUT WHILE TRAVELING

If you have found that most of the restaurants in your area are unable or unwilling to cook for your child (perhaps due to the severity or complexity of her allergies), chances are you will not fare much better with the restaurants at your chosen travel destination. You may want to obtain a restaurant guide for your destination area and contact some restaurants in advance to try to determine if restaurants will be an option. The local Chamber of Commerce or Tourist Information Center for the city you will be visiting may also be able to provide you with a list of local restaurants. See Chapter 9 for a discussion of dining in restaurants.

Sometimes you will find that people will go out of their way to help you. While traveling in the Midwest, Gay and her family went to a small Mexican restaurant. After placing their order, Gay questioned the restaurant owner about the ingredients. She was quite surprised to learn that the restaurant's "secret ingredient" was peanut butter! However, even though it was clear that the family was traveling and would probably never return to his restaurant, the owner insisted on cleaning everything and personally cooking something safe for Ariella... and they all enjoyed a delicious dinner.

When traveling, do not assume that the local outlet of a national or regional restaurant chain will use the same ingredients as the restaurant in your home town. In the South, for instance (the "peanut capital of the U.S."), I have been told that the "vegetable oil" used by many restaurants – including fast food chains – is peanut oil. In California (where I live), soy is usually the "vegetable oil" of choice.

When Raniah moved with her husband and food-allergic toddler from California to South Carolina, she was dismayed to find that many family-style restaurants have peanuts and peanut shells littering the floor. A large bucket of peanuts is placed on each dining table. Diners eat the nuts and throw the shells on the floor!

PREPARING FOOD IN YOUR HOTEL ROOM

Many hotels can provide you with a small refrigerator for your room. When you make your reservations, explain that you will require a refrigerator "for medical reasons." Ask for written confirmation that this refrigerator will be in the room which you have reserved.

COFFEE MAKER CUISINE

Some families get very creative in preparing food using boiling water from the hotel room's coffee maker. Depending on your child's allergies, ideas include:

✦ Instant ramen noodles, minus the seasoning packet if the seasonings look "iffy." You can add soy sauce, margarine, or other seasonings for flavor.

✦ Instant couscous

+ Instant oatmeal or other hot cereal

+ Instant mashed potatoes

BRING AN ELECTRIC SKILLET

Some families bring along an electric skillet and use this to prepare meals in the hotel room. An electric skillet can be used to prepare everything from pancakes to pasta to chicken and more. Just be sure that you set it up on a heat-proof surface (such as a tiled bathroom counter) and that you take extra care to avoid setting off the hotel's smoke alarm!

STAYING IN A ROOM
THAT HAS A KITCHEN

My personal preference is to stay in a motel room that has a kitchenette (or rent a cabin or condominium that has a full kitchen). By preparing all of our food myself I avoid the risks of having our vacation spoiled by an allergic reaction to restaurant food, and I save a great deal of money. Of course, the drawback to this is that it is less of a "vacation" for me because I still have to prepare our meals.

———— ❧ ————

Another option is to prepare your allergic child's meal in your motel kitchenette, and then pack it up and bring it with you to a restaurant that can accommodate the rest of the family. However, as mentioned in chapter 9, not all restaurants will permit you to bring in outside food. If this is what you wish to do, I recommend that you call the restaurant first to verify that you will be allowed to bring food for your allergic child.

WHAT TO BRING

If possible, when planning to prepare food in your room's kitchenette, bring along any hard-to-find food items which you feel are essential to the success of your trip. When you arrive at your destination you can head to the nearest supermarket and/or health food store to purchase everything else.

———— ❧ ————

If you do book a room with a kitchenette, you may want to bring along the following:

❑ A menu plan and grocery list for the food you will be preparing while on vacation.

❑ Any non-perishable food items that are likely to be difficult to find at your destination.

❑ An ice chest or travel refrigerator containing difficult-to-find perishable items (if you are going on a car trip or short plane trip).

❑ A cutting board and a sharp knife.

❑ All of the pots, pans, mixing bowls, utensils, etc., that you will need to prepare your food (or if necessary you can buy inexpensive ones at the supermarket at your destination). Although the motel will probably tell you that the kitchenette is "fully stocked," it may not be – or the items available may not be as clean as you would like them to be.

❑ A fresh sponge, because you do not know what residue is in theirs (or you can purchase one at your destination).

❑ Paper plates and plastic utensils, to cut down on dish washing during your vacation (or you can purchase these at your destination).

❑ Plastic sandwich bags, for use in packing up picnic lunches (or purchase at your destination).

❑ A small ice chest and re-freezable ice packs, for use in packing and carrying picnic lunches.

SAMPLE MENUS

If you are going to be preparing food while on vacation, keep it simple. A sample menu, depending on your child's allergies, may be:

SAMPLE VACATION MENUS	
Breakfast	Cold cereal (with soy milk, rice milk, or cow's milk)
Lunch	Sandwiches, whole fresh fruit, potato chips or tortilla chips
Afternoon Snack	Fruit, carrots, crackers, or chips
Dinner	Pasta and salad OR Hamburgers with canned corn and watermelon OR Pan-fried steak with tomato slices and microwaved baked potatoes
Dessert	Whatever easily-available packaged dessert your child can have

STAYING WITH FRIENDS OR RELATIVES

If you will be staying with friends or relatives at your destination, you will need to make sure that they are fully aware of your child's situation and the many precautions that need to be taken to keep her and her food supply safe (including precautions that need to be taken prior to your arrival).

DISCUSS YOUR CHILD'S NEEDS

When you first start to make travel plans, call your hosts to discuss your child's special needs. When you go, bring this book with you. When you arrive, review the pertinent sections with your hosts.

When Donna and her family were invited to stay at a relative's house, she discussed a number of precautions which she needed them to take in order to keep her son Patrick safe. "Before we come I want you to discuss this with your family," she said to her host, "and be sure that you want us to come. I don't want to impose, but this is what is necessary to make it safe for Patrick." Her requests included the following:

✦ *Clean the house, and wash all tables and counters prior to their arrival.*

✦ *During their visit, do not allow anyone in the house to eat any peanuts or tree nuts; put these products away in a non-visible location.*

✦ *During their visit, prepare only "safe" versions of foods which Patrick could eat, to avoid any confusion regarding which dish was the "safe" version and which was not.*

✦ *During their visit, only use the brand of margarine which is safe for Patrick.*

✦ *During their visit, do not cook eggs or anything which contains eggs.*

Although Donna did not request it, two months prior to their visit her hosts voluntarily stopped eating peanut butter and nuts in the house, and stopped eating anything at all in the family room! Needless to say, Donna and her family had a wonderful visit.

WHAT WILL YOUR CHILD EAT?

Even if you will be staying with friends or relatives at your destination, you will still need to think ahead about what you will be feeding your child. Communicate this to your hosts. No matter how well-meaning they are, your hosts are not likely to know what products are and are not safe for your child. They may even assume that you will all be going out to restaurants for most meals, never realizing how difficult this option can be.

STAYING WITH UNSUPPORTIVE RELATIVES

What do you do if the people you will be staying with are not supportive of your child's special needs? If staying elsewhere or not taking the trip at all are not options, you will need to remain extra-vigilant throughout your visit.

Anjali takes her family on regular visits to see her parents, who are unable to visit her due to her father's poor health. Although she reminds everyone prior to her visit to remove all nut products, scrub countertops, etc., she has found that this just does not get done consistently. Now, she says, she has "lowered all expectations." When she arrives, she checks around in the kitchen and refrigerator. She cleans the tables and countertops as needed. While there she prepares all of Rebecca's food herself, and Rebecca is never left alone with anyone other than Anjali or her husband. It is stressful, but it is necessary to ensure Rebecca's safety during these visits.

OTHER VACATION OPTIONS

RECREATIONAL VEHICLES

Another vacation option is to rent, borrow, or purchase a motor home or recreational vehicle (R.V.). This option provides all the benefits of staying in a room with a kitchenette, and (at least in the United States) is a very popular mode of travel.

───── ❧ ─────

If you are using a rented or borrowed R.V., be sure to thoroughly clean the entire inside prior to your trip, in order to remove any food residue or particles left behind by others. This way you can be confident that the R.V. is a completely "safe" environment for your child.

INTERNATIONAL PERSPECTIVE

COUNTRY	COMMENTS
New Zealand	Motor homes are a relatively common way for international visitors to travel around New Zealand –especially for families and couples.

CRUISES

Some people have had good experiences going on cruises, whereas others have found cruise lines to be very unaccommodating. As with any other vacation, taking your food-allergic child on a cruise requires advance planning. Before booking a cruise, contact the cruise line and explain your situation:

❑ Ask to talk to the head chef, and find out what – if anything – your child would be able to eat on board (see Chapter 9 regarding eating in restaurants).

❑ If the ship's restaurants cannot accommodate your child, would there be a way for you to safely store and heat food that you bring aboard yourself?

❑ Speak to the ship's doctor to find out if he or she is equipped to handle an anaphylactic reaction. After all, you may be far out at sea when your child has a reaction. Make sure the doctor is equipped to do more than just administer your EpiPen®!

❑ If you would like to be able to leave your child in the "children's club" area, find out what can be done to make this a safe environment. At the very least, you need to ensure that during your stay the club does not serve highly allergenic food to the other children, and that you will be able to train the children's club staff to recognize and treat an allergic reaction.

AIR TRAVEL IN GENERAL

BRINGING EPIPENS® ONTO AIRPLANES

If you are going to be traveling by air with your child, you must contact your child's allergist in advance to obtain a written doctor's note permitting you to bring your EpiPens® on board the plane. With today's security regulations, this is a necessity. See Appendix D for a sample document. This document is in addition to the letter from your doctor indicating recommended emergency treatment procedures mentioned earlier in this chapter.

——————✖——————

If you are traveling to a non-English-speaking country you may also want to bring a copy of this letter that has been translated into the local language. This is not a necessity, but it could come in handy if you have any problems with the local security agents.

——————✖——————

It is a good idea to tell the airport baggage screeners about your EpiPens® (and perhaps show them your doctor's letter authorizing you to bring the EpiPens® onto the airplane) **before** you set the EpiPen®-containing fanny pack or luggage onto the x-ray conveyer belt.

Pamela and her husband were "nearly arrested" when their bag full of syringes went through the x-ray machine in Spain without any prior warning being given to the baggage screeners. Luckily they both spoke Spanish and were able to adequately explain the situation and translate the doctor's letter.

BRING EXTRA MEDICINE PACKS AND EPIPENS®

When you travel by air, bring at least two full sets of your child's emergency medication – one to bring on board with you, and one to place in your luggage. For long plane rides (especially those that involve hours spent traveling over an ocean), you need to have more than two EpiPens® on board with you – perhaps up to six. Speak to your child's allergist regarding how many to bring.

In addition, if your child has asthma, be sure to have this medication on board with you, too. If your child uses a nebulizer, you need to bring a portable battery-operated nebulizer onto the airplane.

BRING ALL OF YOUR CHILD'S FOOD

Always bring a lunch box or small cooler containing **all** of the food that your child will need for the trip, including extra food in case you are unexpectedly delayed. Only bring food which your child will enjoy when served cold, such as sandwiches. Bring at least twice as much as you think you need. Have this food on the plane with you.

Pamela recommends bringing small paper bowls or plates and then obtaining plastic utensils from one of the restaurants that is located inside the airport (after you have passed the x-ray machines).

———— ✦ ————

In addition to meals, don't forget to bring along an assortment of ready-to-eat snacks. Have some in your hand luggage, your suit case, your purse, etc. When your children become whiny and hungry you will want to have something convenient to give them to eat (this, of course, is good advice whether or not you're dealing with food allergies!).

———— ✦ ————

Do not permit your child to eat **any** of the food that is served by the airline. Although it might appear to be safe, it is not worth taking risks when you arc milcs up in thc air! Stick with thc food that you brought from home.

Heidi once ordered a "plain fruit bowl" from the airline for her food-allergic daughter, Marlee. When it arrived it looked delicious. Before handing the dish to Marlee, however, Heidi poked it around a bit with a fork. Hiding under the orange segments she found a pile of pecans and walnuts!

———— ✦ ————

Bring bottled water for your child to drink on the airplane. Although the airline can certainly provide water, it is best if the airline personnel do not touch anything which your child will be consuming on the flight.

WEAR LONG PANTS AND LONG SLEEVES

When traveling by air, have your child wear long pants and long sleeves, to minimize the risk of his skin coming in contact with allergens on the trip.

BOOK THE FIRST FLIGHT OF THE DAY

Your chances of flying on an airplane that has been freshly cleaned and vacuumed are greater if you purchase tickets for the first flight of the day.

BOOK A DIRECT FLIGHT

If possible, cut down on potential problems by booking a direct flight. It is easier to get special accommodations on one plane than on two or three planes.

Gay took all of the appropriate precautions prior to her flight with her egg- and peanut-allergic daughter, including making arrangements for a peanut-free flight. Everything went well until they got to their connecting flight. Due to a mechanical problem, there had been a last-minute switch of airplanes on this flight. The new airplane, of course, was not peanut-free.

DON'T SIT NEXT TO STRANGERS

Plan to have your child sit at the window seat, with you or another member of your family next to her. This will reduce her potential exposure to allergens.

IF YOUR CHILD HAS A REACTION ON THE PLANE

If, despite your precautions, your child should have a reaction during the flight, follow your physician's treatment instructions and then immediately notify the flight crew.

AIR TRAVEL FOR THE PEANUT ALLERGIC

Air travel can be especially dangerous for the peanut-allergic. Although some airlines have switched to serving pretzels or other snack items, little bags of roasted peanuts are still ubiquitous on many flights. A danger can be posed when hundreds of little bags of peanuts are opened within a short period of time, causing peanut dust to go into the closed-circuit air system of the plane. In addition, it is a good bet that on peanut-serving airlines, there is a fine layer of peanut dust coating the entire interior of the plane. In addition to the precautions described on pages 119-122, there are additional steps that you should take.

Visit www.foodallergy.org, the website of the Food Allergy and Anaphylaxis Network, for a current list of airlines that do not serve peanut snacks. If possible, book a flight on one of these airlines.

ADVANCE PLANNING TO MINIMIZE RISKS

If you plan to travel by air with your peanut-allergic child on an airline that does regularly serve peanuts, you should do the following to minimize the risks:

❑ Call the airline as far in advance as possible to request that peanuts not be served on your flights. Do not request a "peanut-free" flight. Because the airlines cannot control the food brought on board by other passengers, they cannot promise a "peanut-free flight" and making this request will most likely cause you to run into resistance. The most the airline can do is agree not to serve peanuts.

❏ Keep a record of the date and time you called, the name of the person you spoke to, and the promises made. Ask for written confirmation of the airline's response.

❏ If you are not satisfied with the responses given to you by the first person with whom you speak, insist on talking to his or her supervisor. (And if this person cannot help you, talk to his supervisor, and so on). Do not give up. You are not making an unreasonable request, and you are certainly not the first person to make this request.

❏ Make sure that the airline you are speaking to is the airline that is actually operating the flight. It is possible that the airline through which you booked the flight has some type of agreement with another airline that in fact operates the flight – and there is no guarantee that this other airline will be informed of any special arrangements which you make.

❏ Call the airline again one week before your trip to confirm that there will be no peanuts served on your flights.

❏ Obtain the name and telephone number of the supervisor or special service coordinator to contact in case you have a problem en route.

❏ When you arrive at the check-in counter on the day of your trip, confirm that there will be no peanuts served on your flight.

❏ When you arrive at the gate, re-confirm that there will be no peanuts served on your flight, and explain to the gate personnel that you will need to board the plane in advance of the rush of passengers.

❏ Don't forget to call the airline again before your return flight to confirm that no peanuts will be served.

REMOVING PEANUT RESIDUE
FROM YOUR CHILD'S SEAT AREA

Bring the following items on board with you:

❏ Wet wipes

❏ Wide masking tape

❏ Your child's food and medications

❏ Your doctor's note permitting you to bring your EpiPens® on the plane.

———❧———

You – but preferably not your child – should board the plane when people with special needs are allowed to pre-board. If you are traveling alone with your child, you may need to enlist the help of an airline staff person to watch your child (within your view) at this time. In order to try to remove the layer of peanut dust and other food residue that may be on the seats, you should do the following:

❏ Take a long piece of masking tape and use it like a lint catcher to go over all of the upholstery in your row.

❏ Use 5 or 6 of the wet wipes to wipe down the seats, armrests, seat backs, trays, windows, window area, and all other exposed surfaces in your entire row.

❏ Remove all the magazines and such from the seat back in front of your child's seat, and clean out this area as well.

❏ Throw away the soiled masking tape and wet wipes so they will not contaminate anything.

❏ Check the floor and remove any food particles from this area.

❏ Step into the lavatory to wash your hands with soap.

❏ Bring your child on board.

———❧———

If your child is very sensitive, you should go through this cleaning routine even if you are flying on a "peanut-free" airline. Although in this case the airline itself does not serve peanuts, many passengers (especially children) bring their own snacks and candies on board with them and there is still a risk of allergenic residue on the seats.

KEEP YOUR CHILD IN THE CLEAN SEAT
During the flight, keep your child occupied in your (clean) row. Do not allow him to wander through the airplane.

REPEAT EVERYTHING FOR THE RETURN TRIP
Don't forget to repeat everything – including packing food for your child – for the trip back home.

CHAPTER 11

PRESCHOOL

———❦———

Creating a safe preschool environment for your child is very do-able but will require a great deal of communication and cooperation between you, the preschool staff, and (sometimes) the parents of the other children in the class. The relative ease or difficulty of creating a safe preschool environment for your child will depend largely on the severity of your child's allergies and whether you are signing your child up for a preschool class that only meets a few hours a day (either before or after meal time) or a full day program.

———❦———

Although you may find it difficult to imagine entrusting the care of your food-allergic child to anyone else, let me assure you that thousands (if not millions) of children like yours have successfully and safely attended preschool.

———❦———

Most of the issues relating to creating a safe school environment for an older food-allergic child are pertinent for a younger child as well. In this chapter I have focused primarily on information that is only pertinent to a young child. Because preschool is not mandatory, I have placed the information that is pertinent to all age groups in a separate chapter. Chapter 12, "School," focuses primarily on the elementary school years (with some discussion of junior and senior high school and college as well).

———❦———

Before reading this chapter, I highly recommend that you skip ahead and **read Chapter 12 first.**

**INTERNATIONAL
PERSPECTIVE**

COUNTRY	COMMENTS
United Kingdom	Food allergy-related "Guidance for Preschool" information is posted on the Anaphylaxis Campaign's website, www.anaphylaxis.org.uk.

IF YOUR CHILD IS ALREADY IN PRESCHOOL

If your child's initial food allergy diagnosis takes place after he is already in a preschool or daycare situation, do not be surprised if your current daycare provider is unwilling or uninterested in learning how to keep your child safe.

Tanya's toddler was diagnosed shortly after he had started to be cared for by a new daycare provider. Tanya found this woman's comments about "not getting paid enough for all we're putting her through" or how much they were "driving her crazy" hard to shrug off.

In situations such as this, if your current daycare provider is unable or unwilling to create a safe environment for your child, you must find a new caregiver. Do not endanger your child.

GET ORGANIZED

Before you begin to contact preschools or daycare providers to determine the best placement for your child, get organized. Have a draft of a written emergency action plan (see Appendix B for a sample form) that you can share with the school director. Start a list (not necessarily a complete list) of steps that you feel the school will need to take in order to keep your child safe. Practice clearly articulating the details of your child's special needs. Be able to explain the seriousness of your child's allergies. This advance preparation will help your meetings with school directors to go more smoothly.

LOOK FOR A PRESCHOOL WITH PRIOR FOOD ALLERGY EXPERIENCE

It is to your advantage to find a preschool or daycare provider which has already successfully accommodated severely food-allergic children. If you belong to a food allergy support group, network with the other members to find appropriate facilities in your area.

CONTACT SCHOOL DIRECTORS IN YOUR AREA

Contact the directors of the preschools or the daycare providers in your area to begin a conversation about your child's special needs. Very simply tell them what your child is allergic to, explain the severity of the allergies, and talk to them about some of the steps that you would need them to take to keep your child safe. At the end of this initial telephone call, make an appointment to sit down with the preschool director to discuss your child's placement in much greater detail.

———❦———

If you are told, "Don't worry. We have a number of children at this facility who have food allergies," ask a few more questions before you rejoice at your good fortune. How severe are these other children's allergies? For example, do they have EpiPens® on campus for use in case of an allergic reaction? What special precautions are being taken to keep these children safe? If the answers are that there are no EpiPens® and no special precautions, these other children clearly have much less serious allergies. You will need to explain that your child's situation is quite different.

———❦———

Remember, you must feel good about where you leave your child. If, for example, the preschool director or teacher responds defensively to your questions about class projects and supplies used, this is probably not the best placement for your child. Follow your instincts regarding whether or not a particular preschool is the right one for your family.

ISSUES TO ADDRESS

In addition to the issues presented in Chapter 12, you and the staff also need to address the following:

❑ For some severely peanut-allergic children, the only way to create a safe environment at this age is to create a completely peanut-free facility. Peanut butter is a very sticky substance, and is hard to remove from all the surfaces of the room. It is extremely difficult for the school to ensure that every child who eats a peanut butter sandwich for lunch gets properly washed up immediately thereafter.... before he touches (and contaminates) anything. It is quite likely that your child's classmates would get peanut butter residue in their hair or on their clothing as well. These "contaminated" classmates can be like ticking time bombs for your child.

Is the school willing to accommodate your request for a peanut-free facility – and require all of the other parents to accommodate this as well?

❑ If peanut butter is allowed in the preschool that your peanut-allergic child attends, how will the lunch tables be cleaned? If sponges are used, traces of peanut butter will remain in the sponge. These tables must be washed with disposable cloths. How will the school ensure that the other children are thoroughly cleaned up immediately after they eat? How will they keep the entire facility from becoming contaminated with peanut butter residue?

❑ What steps will be taken to quickly clean up allergenic food which is on or dropped by the other children in the class?

❑ You and the staff need to agree upon a system to ensure that your child's bottle or cup is easily distinguished (by your child, the staff, and the other students) as being hers.

❑ If the facility accommodates very young children who are fed in highchairs, request that the chairs be spaced far enough apart so that the children cannot grab each other's food.

❑ If your child has a wheat allergy, the school should not set out any commercially purchased play dough. Provide the school with a recipe for homemade wheat-free play dough (see Appendix L) or offer to be the one who makes it for the class.

❑ Most preschools have a wide variety of hands-on items in the room for the children to touch and explore. What is on the touch tables, science tables, smell tables, etc.? Popular tactile items that may pose a problem for your child include crab shells, egg shells, beans, rice, and other foods. Work with the teacher to find acceptable alternatives.

KEEP MEDICINE PACK AND EMERGENCY INSTRUCTIONS HANDY

Your child's medicine packs, clearly labeled with your child's name, in brightly colored, well-labeled pouches, should be hanging up high in plain view in the classroom and in whatever other locations throughout the campus that you and the preschool management have agreed upon. Complete emergency instructions (see Appendix B for sample form) should be inside this pack.

———❧———

A laminated one-page sheet containing a picture of your child and a list of her allergies should be posted out of the children's reach in several strategic locations throughout the preschool, such as on the classroom door, at the front office, in the kitchen, and in any areas where food is served. This is meant to serve as a reminder to staff and parents about your child's special needs.

LABEL FOODS AS "SAFE" OR "NOT SAFE"

Even if your child is not going to be eating any of the food supplied by the preschool or daycare center, it is helpful for the staff to know which of their snacks are allergenic for your child and which are not. If they are serving an allergenic food to the rest of the class, they will know to be extra careful with the clean-up. Make arrangements to go into the center's kitchen once or twice a week (depending on how frequently they purchase food supplies) and apply the same "red and green dot" food marking system which you may be using in your own home (see page 51).

ONLY GIVE YOUR CHILD FOOD WHICH YOU HAVE APPROVED

Remember, when an adult gives a young child something to eat, the young child will respect the adult's knowledge and authority and assume that the food must be safe. Therefore you should instruct the school staff that they are only to give your child food which you brought in or which you personally approved.

SERVE YOUR CHILD'S FOOD ON A CAFETERIA TRAY

Purchase a large plastic cafeteria-style tray (with a raised edge) and ask your child's preschool or daycare center to serve her lunch on this tray. Children of this age are very messy eaters. This will help protect your child's food from her classmates' inevitable lunchtime and snack time spills. Discuss with the staff who will be responsible for cleaning this tray each day.

WHEN PARENTS TAKE TURNS BRINGING SNACKS

In many preschool programs, the parents take turns bringing in snacks for all of the children in the class. If this is the case, there are three main options for how to handle snacks:

SNACK OPTION	OPTION'S DRAWBACKS
You bring a separate snack for your child.	The other children's snack may pose a danger to your child.
You distribute a list of "safe" snacks, described by brand name and variety, and all of the parents agree to only bring snacks that are on this list (and you also bring an "emergency back-up" snack for your child just in case the wrong item is accidentally purchased).	This only works if your child's allergies are not so restrictive as to make it impossible to create a reasonable list of commonly available snack foods. Also, there is a risk that ingredients will change between the time you create your list and the time another parent buys the item, or that a parent will buy the wrong brand or variety of a listed item.
The parents all pay a "snack fee," and you commit to purchasing and bringing ALL of the snacks every time.	This is a huge commitment on your part, and it deprives the other children in the class of the fun of being the snack person

Michelle's son attends a "mornings only" preschool program which does not include lunch. Although the school usually takes responsibility for providing snacks for the children, Michelle made arrangements for her to purchase all of the snacks for the entire class, with the school reimbursed her for her expenses. This way Michelle was able to ensure that only "safe" snacks were served. In addition, a letter was sent to the other parents explaining the situation, and requesting that only non-food treats be sent to school for classroom birthday celebrations.

FOOD ALLERGY BOOKS AND VIDEOS FOR PRESCHOOLERS

FAAN has some wonderful videos and books designed to teach very young children and their classmates about food allergies. "Alexander, the Elephant Who Couldn't Eat Peanuts," for example, is an excellent video to show in a preschool or Kindergarten classroom. It features a brief cartoon followed by a segment showing a variety of young children talking about their allergies. They have also produced an entire series of children's books aimed at this age group.

 INTERNATIONAL PERSPECTIVE

COUNTRY	COMMENTS
New Zealand	Allergy New Zealand has education kits designed both for preschools and schools. Go to www.allergy.org.nz to download the resource order form. Many of FAAN's resources are available here as well.
United Kingdom	The Anaphylaxis Campaign has also produced children's books and videos. Visit www.anaphylaxis.org.uk for details..

NOTES

CHAPTER 12

SCHOOL AND DAY CARE

Depending on the severity of your child's allergies, creating a safe school environment for your food-allergic child can be a persistent challenge, especially in a public school setting. On-going cooperation and communication between you and your child's teacher, principal, school nurse, and other school staff members is a necessity.

Unfortunately, there is no "one size fits all" approach to managing food allergies in a school setting. The appropriate measures to take and procedures to implement depend on the type and severity of your child's allergies, your child's age, how food is usually handled by the particular school, and a host of other variables. The information provided in this section is meant as a guideline to make you aware of many of the potential issues and possible solutions for creating a safe school environment for your child. Depending on the severity of your child's allergies, many of the issues raised in this chapter may not be relevant for your child.

 INTERNATIONAL PERSPECTIVE

COUNTRY	COMMENTS
Canada	Anaphylaxis Canada's website contains a detailed information section for schools and camps, including a sample school policy, handbook for school boards, lesson plans, and more. Visit www.anaphylaxis.ca for details.

INTERNATIONAL PERSPECTIVE, *CONTINUED*

COUNTRY	COMMENTS
United Kingdom	For information specifically pertinent to school children in the U.K., see the Anaphylaxis Campaign's booklet, "Anaphylaxis and Schools: How We Can Make It Work." The information contained in this booklet is also posted on the group's website, www.anaphylaxis.org.uk. In addition, a government document entitled "Supporting Pupils with Medical Need" is available from the Department for Education and Skills (DFES) publication division. Telephone 0845 6022260.

BEFORE- AND AFTER-SCHOOL DAYCARE

If your child will be attending an onsite or offsite before- or after-school daycare center, all of the issues raised in this chapter must be addressed with the daycare center operators as well.

YOUR CHILD'S LEGAL RIGHTS

In the United States, food-allergic children cannot be denied attendance at public school. A child's right to be accommodated by the public school system is guaranteed by federal law.

INTERNATIONAL
PERSPECTIVE

COUNTRY	COMMENTS
Australia	A food-allergic child cannot be denied attendance at a public school, although it is discretionary for private schools.
Canada	Canadian children have a right to a safe education in the public schools system. Schools have a legal duty to accommodate children with physical disabilities, although this duty can be limited by the principal of undue (financial) hardship.
New Zealand	All children between the age of 5 and 19 have a right to attend school and receive an education (section 3 Education Act 1989). As with students with many medical conditions, food-allergic students cannot be denied their right to an education.
United Kingdom	The Anaphylaxis Campaign believes that children with severe food allergies are covered by the Special Educational Needs and Disability Act. This Act says that disabled pupils must not be treated less favorably, without justification, than other pupils, and that schools must make reasonable adjustments to ensure that they are not put to any substantial disadvantage. In addition, under this Act it is likely to be unlawful for any school to refuse to let staff members volunteer to administer medicine to allergic pupils – and the head teacher would be obliged to find volunteers to undertake this responsibility. School trips and after-school activities are also covered by this legislation.

TALK TO SCHOOL PERSONNEL
IN ADVANCE OF THE SCHOOL YEAR

Months before the start of the school year you should make an appointment to sit down with the appropriate school personnel (such as principal, classroom teacher, and nurse) to discuss a myriad of issues relevant to creating a safe and inclusive school environment for your child.

PREPARE FOR THE MEETING

Prior to your meeting with the school administration, create a simple one-page Food Allergy Action Plan which explains how to recognize and treat an allergic reaction (see Appendix B). Although your school may have additional forms and paperwork for you to fill out, it is good to arrive at the meeting prepared with this vital information.

———————

In addition, you need to do an honest assessment (based on your prior experience and your physician's advice) of the severity of your child's allergies. Does he react to airborne particles? Does he react to things which he touches? Can he be trusted to keep his fingers out of his mouth, nose and eyes? Does he react to food which has merely touched a small amount of allergen? Or does he only react if he takes a bite of an allergenic food? The answers to these questions will help determine what measures will need to be taken in order to keep your child safe.

———————

At this meeting, make it a point to be friendly, organized, and enthusiastically positive. Your "can-do" attitude and obvious helpfulness will help create a positive atmosphere and help to allay any fears that the staff may have about your child's needs.

———————

Choose your words carefully. Use phrases such as "let's do...," "we'll need to...," or "we should plan for...," instead of "you should," "you will," or "you must." Be positive in your approach.

PUT EVERYTHING IN WRITING

After your meeting, put the agreed-upon food allergy management plan in writing. This will remind everyone what was agreed upon and provide an opportunity for misunderstandings to be resolved.

ISSUES TO ADDRESS

Your discussion with the school staff should address the following:

EMERGENCY TRAINING

❏ Who will be responsible for training classroom teachers, special-subject teachers, lunchroom and playground monitors, first aid clerks, janitors, school bus drivers and other school personnel regarding your child's special needs and the steps that must be taken if your child has an allergic reaction while at school (or on the way to or from school)?

 **INTERNATIONAL
PERSPECTIVE**

COUNTRY	COMMENTS
United Kingdom	In the U.K., the school nurse usually is responsible for conducting this training. The Anaphylaxis Campaign's "Action for Anaphylaxis" video is suitable for use during these training sessions.

❏ Who will be trained? Request that the **entire** staff be trained to recognize and treat your child's allergic reactions. It is not sufficient to limit this training to the classroom teacher or the school nurse. You cannot count on this one person being available at the exact moment that your child has a reaction. You want the entire staff to be "on board" the program to keep your child safe and alive. Plus, some people (possibly one of your child's teachers) simply do not think clearly during an emergency.

❏ What will be included in this training session? As part of this training, procedures need to be implemented that will enable the staff to recognize your child's symptoms as being a potential allergic reaction and not a sudden illness. For example, if your child vomits in the lunch area, the staff must assess whether this is an allergic reaction or a flu.

❏ When will the first training session be held? It is not acceptable for the training to take place after your child's first day of school.

❏ How often will these training sessions take place? It is desirable to have an initial training session prior to the start of the school year, and "refresher courses" two weeks later and at mid-term. As the school year goes on, it is easy for the school staff to be lulled into a false sense of security, especially if they have been doing such a good job that your child does not have any allergic reactions while at school.

❏ Who will be responsible for ensuring that substitute teachers receive this same training before they begin the school day in your child's classroom? What will be the protocol for making sure that this takes place?

❏ Who will be responsible for training personnel who are hired after the initial training session is held?

❏ Many schools have special teams of personnel who have been trained to take charge in the event of a catastrophe (such as a bio-terrorist attack, an earthquake, a school lockdown, and so forth). In the event of a catastrophe they will wear hard hats, conduct searches for missing children in the dark, provide medications to at-risk children, and perform other such emergency duties. This team needs to know who your child is, where her medication is kept, and how to recognize and treat an allergic reaction.

LOCATION OF MEDICINE PACKS

❑ Where will your child's emergency medication be kept?

❑ Will it be easily accessible from the classroom, lunch area and playground?

❑ Is the school aware that the medication should not be stored in a refrigerator?

❑ Is it school policy to keep all medications locked in a cupboard? If so, this is not acceptable. In an emergency, your child could die in the time it will take the school office personnel to locate the key, unlock the cupboard, and find the medication. It is imperative that your child's medication be kept in readily accessible locations.

❑ How many sets of emergency medication will be kept on campus? For example, you may need one in the classroom, one in the lunch area, one in the office, one in the playground aides' backpack, one in the classroom teacher's emergency backpack which is taken with the class during an evacuation, and one in the disaster team's emergency supply area. In some schools, medications are kept in a fanny pack that is handed from one teacher or aide to the next as the child moves through the school.

❑ Emphasize that the storage location(s) of your child's medicine kit(s) must remain constant and easily accessible. School personnel must be able to easily find the kit in an emergency. If there are situations for which the medication will be moved from its storage location (such as for field trips), there must be a system in place to ensure that it gets returned to its proper place.

ALLOWING CHILD TO CARRY MEDICINE PACK

❑ For older children, it is often best to have the child wear a fanny pack containing the emergency medication. What are your school's policies regarding this?

SCHOOL BUS ISSUES

❑ If your child is transported to and from school on a school bus, will there be an additional medicine pack that is kept on the bus (and is it always physically the same bus that is used in the morning as in the afternoon)?

❏ What rules or procedures need to put in place (such as a "no eating food on the bus" policy) to ensure your child's safety while on the school bus?

CREATING A SAFE CLASSROOM ENVIRONMENT

Creating a safe classroom environment allows the teacher to focus on teaching rather than worrying about your child.

❏ What steps will the school take to ensure a safe and allergen-free classroom? Suggestions include:

✦ Banning food from the classroom itself (perhaps the class can go into a different room for snacks, celebrations, and other food-eating occasions).

✦ Having each child thoroughly wipe his or her hands with a wet wipe prior to entering the classroom in the morning, after snack or recess, and after lunch (you may have to supply these wet wipes) – or, if there is a sink available near the classroom door, having each child wash his or her hands with soap.

✦ Removing allergen-containing projects from the lesson plans.

✦ If your child's class contains "hands on" materials, ensuring that these materials are allergen-free as well.

❏ If your child is contact sensitive to allergens, find out if the children commonly share supplies (such as pencils, scissors, and rulers) in the classroom. If they do, you should arrange to supply a separate set of materials just for your child, which no one else will be allowed to touch or use.

❏ Will your child's classroom have any class pets? If so, are there any allergenic ingredients in the pets' food? If your child is also allergic to animals, can the pet be removed from the classroom?

❏ Your child's classroom should not be used for any after school activities, such as Scout meetings, at which snacks may be served.

❏ If your child is extremely sensitive to particular allergens, make sure that your child's teacher understands that it is not safe for him to even touch foods which contain these allergens. Many teachers like to use food products for math lessons, art projects, and so forth. Work together with the teacher to find safe substitutes that can be used for the **whole** class. Do not agree to let your child use a "safe" material while the rest of the class uses an allergenic material. This will create an unsafe classroom situation and will isolate your child.

FOOD BROUGHT INTO THE CLASSROOM

❑ What will be the policy regarding food brought in for classroom parties and celebrations?

❑ What about food (such as candy) that is in "goody bags" that other parents bring in as part of birthday celebrations?

❑ What will be the policy regarding food brought in for classroom cultural presentations? Many schools encourage parents to make these presentations. Who will communicate this policy to the parents?

EXPLAINING YOUR CHILD'S FOOD ALLERGIES TO HIS CLASSMATES

❑ How will your child's allergies be explained to the other children in the classroom?

❑ Will the teacher or nurse give this explanation, or will you come into the classroom to give a presentation? After the age of 9 or 10, it is best if this information be presented by the school nurse, in a way that will not single your child out. **Note:** Some excellent resources are available to help explain food allergies to younger children.

YOUR CHILD'S FOOD

❑ If the school cafeteria is to provide food for your child, who will be responsible for ensuring that the ingredients used are "allergen-free" and that the food has not been contaminated with allergens during the preparation or serving process?

❑ Where will your child eat lunch and snack?

❑ How will your child be kept safe during lunch and snack times? (See pages 143-148 for a discussion about creating a safe lunch environment.)

"PEANUT-FREE" POLICIES

❑ Will the school be enacting a "no peanuts" policy, "peanut-free lunch table" or other such program? If so, how will it be enforced?

❑ If you are requesting a "peanut-free classroom" you must clearly articulate what you mean by "peanut-free." The school personnel might think that this merely means that the teacher will not plan any activities that involve peanuts. Make sure it is understood that "peanut-free" means that no one brings anything which contains peanuts into the classroom under any circumstances (including snacks, party foods, crafts, lunches, etc.).

❑ If you are going to have a "peanut-free classroom," a letter needs to be sent from the school administration to the parents of your child's classmates explaining the policy. See Appendix G for a sample letter explaining sample food allergy policies. It is important that this letter be sent from the school principal or nurse rather than from you.

"NO FOOD SHARING" POLICIES

❏ Is the school willing to enact – and enforce – a school wide "no food sharing or trading" policy?

HAND WASHING POLICIES

❏ Is there a way to ensure that the other children wash their hands after eating, especially before they leave the lunch area to go to the playground? Keep in mind that "instant hand sanitizers" do not provide an adequate method for removing food residue.

SAFETY ON THE PLAYGROUND

❏ How will your child be kept safe on the playground (especially if the other children did not wash their hands in between lunch and recess)?

KEEPING "SAFE" FOOD ON CAMPUS

❏ Where can you keep a supply of safe non-perishable snacks and treats at school for your child?

❏ Where can you keep a safe non-perishable "emergency lunch" for your child to eat in case her lunch becomes contaminated when one of her classmates spills their food or drink? This lunch can include safe canned fruit, canned meat (such as tuna), crackers, etc. Don't forget to include a can opener!

❏ Who should your child notify if she needs this lunch?

FOOD FOR EMERGENCIES

❏ If your school stores food supplies to be used by the students during an emergency (such as after an earthquake or during a storm), find out exactly what is being provided. Make sure, for example, that in a city-wide emergency your peanut-allergic child will not be surrounded by a school full of children eating peanut butter. Also, make arrangements for you to provide appropriate emergency food supplies for your child, clearly labeled as being only for your child.

❏ What does your school's cafeteria serve as an "emergency back-up" if the power goes out? Just as in the earthquake/storm scenario, you do not want your peanut-allergic child surrounded by an entire school full of children eating peanut butter. If peanut butter sandwiches are what would normally be served in this situation, suggest that the school plans to serve jam sandwiches instead.

Keeping Change of Clothing on Campus

❏ Where can you keep a full change of clothing for your child, to be used in case something allergenic is spilled on him? After your child reaches middle school or junior high, the clothes he keeps at school for physical education class can do "double duty" for this purpose.

Physical Education Class

❏ Who will ensure that the medicine pack is taken to physical education class – and returned to its proper place afterward?

Fire Drills and Field Trips

❏ Who will be responsible for taking your child's medication with the class during fire drills, field trips, and other times when the class will be leaving the school building?

❏ How will your child be kept safe on field trips – both on the bus ride and while at the destination? When your child participates in a school field trip, his medication pack must travel in the vehicle with him. For instance, if he's traveling in a school bus and the teacher is in a separate car, the medicine, and an adult who knows how and when to use it, needs to be on the bus. Once at the destination, your child's group needs to be escorted throughout the field trip by an adult who has and knows how and when to use the emergency medication.

Lessons and Art Projects Using Food or Food Containers

❏ Many popular children's art projects involve the use of empty food containers (such as milk cartons and egg cartons). Explain to your child's teacher that these containers must be **thoroughly** washed in hot soapy water prior to being brought into the classroom.

❏ Many popular school projects include food items, such as math lessons using dry cold cereal; dry pasta, bean, lentil, and seed collages; pasta necklaces; art projects using empty nut shells (such as "turtles" made out of walnut shell halves); collages using broken pieces of dried colored egg shells; and more. Alert your child's teacher to the potential dangers of these types of projects.

"Housekeeper" Duties

❏ At many schools the children rotate through lunch table cleaning duties and classroom "housekeeper" duties. Find out if this is the case at your child's school. Your child should not be permitted to have these jobs.

COOKING CLASSES

❏ If cooking instruction is part of the curriculum, will your child be allowed to participate? If so, you need to work with the cooking teacher to ensure that all ingredients used are completely safe, that wooden utensils are not used (they may have absorbed allergenic oils used in prior cooking projects) and that the teacher is watching out for allergenic residue in the kitchen (such as on the work surface, on the pots and pans, etc.) left by other classes.

❏ If your child will not be participating, what will he be doing while the other children are cooking?

CREATING A SAFE LUNCH ENVIRONMENT

Creating a safe lunch environment in a school setting for a severely food-allergic child is very problematic, especially for those with peanut allergy. Peanut allergy is considered to be the most lethal of the common food allergies; people have died after consuming a quantity of peanut that could best be described as a "crumb." In the United States, peanut butter is ubiquitous at lunch time, and hard-to-clean-off peanut butter residue is therefore ubiquitous in most school lunch areas. Luckily the problem does improve in the junior and senior high years, as teens and pre-teens usually eat their food quite neatly, without spreading food residue all around.

In striving to create a safe lunch environment for your child, your goal should be to minimize the likelihood of an allergic reaction, while ensuring that the school personnel are completely prepared to recognize and treat a reaction if it should occur.

ASSESS YOUR CHILD'S NEEDS

Depending on the severity of your child's allergies, there may literally be no truly "good" way in which to create a safe environment. Before you talk to the school personnel to work out the best solution possible under your particular circumstances, you need to give some thought to the following questions (and possibly discuss them with your child's physician as well):

✦ Just how severe are my child's food allergies?

✦ Will my child react to airborne particles of an allergen? If your child has multiple food allergies, is this the case for each allergen or just certain ones? For example, assuming the food would not touch her in any way, could your child sit next to a child who was eating a peanut butter sandwich?

✦ Will my child only react if she ingests an allergen – and if so, how minute a quantity of allergen is likely to trigger a reaction? For example, if my child touches a tiny amount of food residue on the lunch table and then touches her own sandwich, will she react to the sandwich? Once again, if your child has multiple food allergies, is this the case for each allergen or just certain ones?

✦ Does my child have the awareness and the maturity to notice and respond if another child spills or splatters (possibly allergenic) food on her food or her body?

The answers to these questions will help you to determine what special accommodations your child will require.

POSSIBLE SOLUTIONS

All of the options for creating a reasonably safe lunch environment for your child have associated drawbacks. Here I will present some of the possible solutions, and a discussion of the possible drawbacks of each. In most cases, the "allergen" being avoided is peanuts, even if the child has multiple allergies in addition to peanut allergy. For most food-allergic children, it is only necessary to take "extreme" measures to avoid being near peanuts and tree nuts.

SOLUTION	DESCRIPTION	DRAWBACKS
School-wide peanut ban.	Peanuts and peanut products are completely banned from the school; no one is allowed to bring anything containing peanuts on to campus; peanuts are not served by the school cafeteria.	**Difficult to enforce.** Who will check the ingredients of every item brought by every child? **Causes hostility.** Other parents and children resent being told what to do. **Causes false sense of security,** especially if the child has multiple food allergies. There is a continued need for safety protocols and vigilance anyway. **Sets a precedent.** What is the school supposed to do when other children have extremely severe allergies to other allergens? It is not practical for the school to ban peanuts, milk, eggs, wheat, soy....
Eat somewhere else.	Your child, and a friend who has brought an allergen-free lunch, eat somewhere other than the lunch area (such as in the office or the library). Adult supervision, of course, is provided.	**Social isolation.** Your child misses out on eating with the other children. **Social embarrassment.** Your child is singled out as the "allergy child."
Eat at "allergen-free" table.	The school creates a special table within the regular lunch area where only those children who have brought an "allergen-free" lunch are allowed to eat. In most cases this is a "peanut-free" table. This table is maintained as an "allergen-free" table throughout the day, even during other lunch periods.	**May not be safe.** Sitting with the other children may create a high level of risk for your child. **Social embarrassment.** Your child may be embarrassed by the placement (this is usually the case for older children, but not necessarily true for younger children).

POSSIBLE SOLUTIONS, *CONTINUED*

SOLUTION	DESCRIPTION	DRAWBACKS
Eat at end seat at regular lunch table, possibly with disposable placemat set at your child's place.	Your child eats at the regular table. She is at the end seat, so she can easily get up and leave the table if there is a spill or other problem. For a younger child, a disposable paper placemat is used to prevent her hands or her food from touching the table.	**May not be safe.** Sitting with the other children may create a high level of risk for your child. **Social embarrassment.** Your child may be embarrassed by the placement (this is usually the case for older children, but not necessarily true for younger children).
Hire an aide whose job is to watch your child during lunch.	Regardless of where your child eats, there is an adult hovering nearby whose sole job is to watch over your child.	**Expense.** This is a very expensive option, and your school may not be able to afford it. **Social embarrassment.** Your child is singled out as the one who has such a problem that he requires someone to "hover over him." **Psychological problems.** Your child may develop psychological problems caused by knowing that he has such a serious problem that he requires someone to "hover over him."
No special accommodtions are made.	Your child eats wherever she wants, just like the other children.	**May not be safe.** Sitting with the other children may create a high level of risk for your child.

Keep in mind that your child's lunchtime arrangements are likely to change as he and his classmates get older. For example, in first grade your child may eat lunch with a designated friend in the school office; in second through fourth grades he may progress to eating at a special peanut-free table in the school lunch area; in fifth grade he may eat at the edge seat of a regular lunch table; and by seventh grade he may not have any special lunchtime accommodations. Of course, each child's needs must be evaluated on an individual basis.

You are probably wondering, "So how did Linda handle the lunch issue for her child?" Unfortunately, my answer may not be of much help to you, but here it is:

✦ *In preschool and Kindergarten, Jason was in morning-only programs that did not include lunch.*

✦ *For 1ˢᵗ through 6ᵗʰ grades, Jason attended a private school that does not have a cafeteria or a lunch area. The children eat in the classroom, at their individual desks, with the classroom teacher in the room supervising (one teacher, twenty children). It is the school's policy that the children all wash their hands before they eat, and clean their desks (and, if necessary, the floor around their desks) after they eat. With Jason in attendance we added a rule that all children were to wash their hands after eating as well. Jason had his own sponge, and no one else was permitted to eat at his desk. During the earlier years he was given a desk that was set perpendicular to the other desks in the table grouping (so that no one was sitting directly on either side of him). His classroom was not used for any after-school extra-curricular activities.*

✦ *For 7ᵗʰ grade Jason attended a large (1,500 students in two grades) public Middle School. The school schedule does not have any "recess" or "snack" breaks prior to lunch. The lunch area is outdoors, and it is cleaned at the end of each day. Jason was assigned to the first lunch break so that he would be eating at a relatively clean table. He brought his lunch every day (he kept it in his backpack), and he avoided allowing his food to touch anything other than the containers in which he brought it. He reported that his friends ate their own food very neatly, and spills were not an issue. In case of emergency, Jason wore a fanny pack containing his medicine, which he was authorized to self-administer. Luckily this was not necessary.*

✦ *As I write this, Jason is about to enter 8ᵗʰ grade at the same school. Next year he will be in High School, and I hope that he will continue to be able to eat in the lunch area with the rest of the students.*

BUY A LUNCH BOX THAT OPENS FLAT

It is a good idea to buy a lunch box for your child that opens flat, and to then instruct your child to eat her food directly out of the lunch box.

CLEANING YOUR CHILD'S LUNCH TABLE

If the school has created an allergen-free table (such as a peanut-free table) for your child, you need to talk to the janitor about how this table will be kept clean. It is important that the table not be wiped down with the cloth or the pail of cleaning solution that is used to clean the other tables, as these items may contain allergenic food residue.

> *Gail's daughter Sara eats her lunch at a special peanut-free table. Each day this table is cleaned using a fresh cloth and a fresh pail of bleach solution.*

Even if your child eats at one of the regular lunch tables, it is likely that she and her friends will settle into a routine of eating at a particular table. Speak to the janitor about keeping this particular table "extra clean."

ASK THE SCHOOL NOT TO SERVE PEANUT PRODUCTS

Regardless of what else you implement, if your child is allergic to peanuts there will be a big reduction in risk if the school cafeteria does not serve peanut butter or peanut products. Your school may not be willing to make this accommodation, but it does not hurt to ask!

AVOID LUNCH MIX-UPS

If you are packing school lunches for more than one child, take precautions to avoid mixing up the food-allergic child's lunch with her siblings' lunches. Buy each child a different colored lunch box, and clearly mark the child's name on the top of the box. Double-check the contents of the box before you close it up. As an extra precaution, instruct your children to speak up (before eating) if it appears that they have received the wrong lunch!

HELP THE SCHOOL PERSONNEL TO CREATE A SAFE AND POSITIVE EXPERIENCE

It is not realistic to expect the staff at your child's school to create a safe and positive school experience for your child without your help. You, the school personnel, and, as appropriate, your child need to work together to make this happen.

COMMUNICATION IS THE KEY

Communication and teamwork is really the key to success. Aim to have regular communication with the teacher, staff, nurse, and special subjects teachers (such as the art and science teachers). Do whatever you can to help the school personnel create a safe and inclusive environment for your child.

YOU CAN DO IT

Although the list of issues which must be considered in order to create a safe school environment for your child may seem daunting to both you and the school personnel, you need to maintain a positive "this is do-able" attitude. Remember, there are many other severely food-allergic children out there who are safely attending school.

As the director of Michelle's son's preschool said at the end of Nicholas' first year there, "Food allergies are difficult but do-able, if we all work together."

BRING YOUR CHILD'S PHOTO TO TRAINING SESSIONS

When your principal or school nurse schedules a session at which to teach school personnel about your child's special needs, bring along an 8" x 10" photo of your child. Set the picture in plain view at the front of the room, so everyone can see what your child looks like.

———————

If you have non-allergic but similar-looking children at the same school, it may be helpful to also show pictures of them (as in, "here's the child with food allergies, and here's his brother who looks 'just like him' but doesn't have food allergies").

HAVE A ONE-ON-ONE MEETING WITH THE TEACHER

Try to have a one-on-one meeting with your child's teacher prior to the start of the school year to calm her fears and to emphasize that you want to work with her as a team to create a safe, inclusive school experience for your child. If she has truly understood the severity of your child's allergies she will probably be somewhat hesitant to assume responsibility for his care. If she has not grasped the gravity of the situation, now is your chance to try again to help her to "get it."

I spoke with one of my son's elementary school teachers, and she suggested the following advice for teachers who will have a severely food-allergic child in their classroom: "It's all about overcoming your fear. Encourage the child's parents to share *openly and to teach you exactly what to do in the event of an allergic reaction. Keep a guide which contains this information posted in your classroom, along with all of the medications which may be necessary. Practice until you are confident. Get to know the child and work as a team. You will be ready and yes, **you can do it!**"*

VOLUNTEER TO CLEAN THE CLASSROOM SUPPLIES

Volunteer to come in to the classroom prior to the first day of school to clean all of the classroom supplies. Not only will this allow you to personally see that all classroom materials are free of food residue, this will also give you a chance to look through all materials to be sure that they are safe for your child. And it can be a big help to the teacher.

MEET WITH THE TEACHER AGAIN AFTER SCHOOL STARTS

Meet again with your child's teacher after the first week or two of school, to get an update as to how things are going and if there are any changes that need to be made.

GET INVOLVED

Get involved at your child's school. Make it a point to meet the teachers, staff, and administration. If at all possible, volunteer to help in the classroom, on field trips, and as "room parent." While you're on campus you can work to raise awareness of food allergy issues.

MEET THE SCHOOL'S STAFF

Get to know the recess and lunchroom aides. They are the ones who will be watching out for your child during the most food-filled portions of the day. Meet the school janitor. He or she will be responsible for keeping your child's lunch table "extra clean." Remember these staff members with small gifts and thank you notes during "teacher appreciation week" and throughout the year.

PROVIDE POSITIVE FEEDBACK TO THE SCHOOL PERSONNEL

Provide positive feedback, praise and encouragement to the school staff whenever appropriate. Don't limit your communications to negative issues!

Remember, taking on the responsibility of caring for your child can be very frightening for the school staff. Gail commented that it took her daughter's teacher a few months to realize that Sara was "not some monster that was going to explode on her!" Positive experiences and positive feedback will help build everyone's confidence and good feelings about the situation.

———— ❧ ————

In order to care for your child, your child's teacher has taken on an extra load of responsibility. Show your appreciation with thank you notes and little gifts such as flowers, plants, coffee mugs, tickets to the movies, etc.

In addition to regularly sending notes, flowers, and so forth, at the end of each school year Heidi likes to show her appreciation by preparing a dinner for the teacher to take home and enjoy with her family. Of course, she first inquires as to any special dietary limitations that the teacher may have!

YOUR CHILD'S RESPONSIBILITIES

Teach your child that she should never share or trade snacks or lunches with other children while at school. Explain to her that she may not know exactly what ingredients are in the other child's food, or what other foods may have touched it while it was being prepared. Items that look "just like" the safe ones that you purchase may in fact be a different brand or variety that is not safe. Teach your child to only eat or touch food which you or another designated adult has approved.

———— ❧ ————

Make sure that your child knows who to go to if she believes she is having an allergic reaction, or if she thinks that she ate something (accidentally or otherwise) that may contain an allergen. Role-play what she should do and say in these situations.

———— ❧ ————

If your child wears a fanny pack with her medication, it is her responsibility to keep this fanny pack on at all times – and to remember to put it on before leaving the house in the morning.

Lauralyn keeps a note which says "Fanny Pack" posted on the back of the front seat of her car, right where her daughter Kelly will see it.

IF YOUR CHILD HAS A REACTION AT SCHOOL

Explain to the appropriate school personnel that you need to be contacted at the slightest sign of an allergic reaction. Of course, the school should first treat your child with the appropriate medication – and if your child is having an anaphylactic reaction they should call the rescue squad before they call you. But (especially in the case of a milder reaction) you need to be brought into the loop, so you can help assess the severity of the reaction in order to help the school personnel develop a point of reference. A full discussion of this reaction will help everyone to prevent or be better prepared to handle the next reaction.

——— ❧ ———

After your child has an allergic reaction while at school – especially after a severe reaction – you need to sit down with the appropriate school personnel to calmly discuss the reaction, determine what went wrong, and work together to ensure that the situation does not happen again in the future. During this meeting, do not "attack" the school staff, and do not be critical or accusatory in your questioning. You are a team. The situation is as frightening for them as it is for you, and you need to assume that they fully understand their responsibility and liability. If you are accusatory the school will not want to deal with you, and you will not be as successful in reaching your goal of creating a safe environment for your child.

UPDATE EMERGENCY INSTRUCTIONS ANNUALLY

The written emergency instructions which your school has on file should include a photo of your child. Be sure to review this information and update it with a fresh photo each year!

DO A MEDICINE PACK "SPOT CHECK"

Periodically check the emergency medicine kits that you have stored at your child's school. Do the appropriate personnel know where it is? Is it where it's supposed to be? Have any of the medications expired? Has any of the information changed on any of the paperwork which you have included in the kit?

Once when I asked to see Jason's medicine kit so that I could check the expiration date on the EpiPens®, I was shocked (and livid) when it took close to 10 minutes for it to be located. As it turns out, a substitute P.E. teacher had failed to return the medicine kit to its proper place after a class trip to a neighborhood park. Had this been an actual emergency....

DOUBLE-CHECK EMERGENCY CONTACT INFORMATION

Double-check to be sure that the school has your correct emergency contact information on file.

Heidi was dismayed when she discovered that all of the emergency contact numbers which she had diligently entered onto the school's paperwork (home number, work number, cell phone number, husband's work and cell phone number, etc.) had not been entered into the school's computer system. When an actual emergency took place, Heidi's friend was contacted because the school could not reach Heidi at home. Others in my support group have double-checked this information, only to discover that a typographical error was made when the numbers were entered into the school's computer system.

EPIPEN® TRAINERS

If you leave an EpiPen® Trainer at school or with others, attach a sturdy tag to it which says in large, bright letters "NOT AN EPIPEN." Insist that the trainer be stored in a separate location from the actual medication. Do not allow the trainer to be stored in the medicine pack.

BIRD FEEDERS MADE WITH PEANUT BUTTER

A popular project in many schools (especially preschool and kindergarten) is to make bird feeders by covering something (such as an empty toilet paper tube) with peanut butter, and then rolling the object in bird seed. Inform your peanut-allergic child's teacher that a safe alternative is to substitute pure vegetable shortening for the peanut butter. In addition, many varieties of bird seed contain nuts, whey (a milk derivative), wheat, and other things that your child may be allergic to. It is therefore imperative that you also check the ingredient label on the bird seed package.

IMPLEMENT THE "PAL" PROGRAM

The Food Allergy and Anaphylaxis Network has developed a program for elementary school students called "Be A PAL: Protect A Life from Food Allergies." This educational awareness program is designed to provide educators with information for teaching students about food allergies and to help them learn how to help friends who have food allergies. The PAL materials are available for free at FAAN's website, www.foodallergy.org. Talk to your child's teacher about implementing the PAL program at your child's school.

BENEFITS OF EDUCATING THE ENTIRE CLASS ABOUT FOOD ALLERGIES

During the elementary school years, it is usually best to educate the entire class – each year – about food allergies. A positive benefit of this is that by teaching children tolerance about food allergies you help teach them tolerance in general.

> *During her daughter Ariella's 6th grade year, the school principal and many of the teachers remarked to Gay that this 6th grade class as a whole (most of whom had been at this school with Ariella for seven years) was much more tolerant, compassionate, and caring than any class in the school's history. They attributed this to the fact that for seven years these children had been asked to be tolerant of someone with differences.*

THANK CLASSMATES FOR THEIR COOPERATION

If the other children in your child's class have been asked not to bring certain foods to school, it is important for your family to thank and acknowledge these classmates' cooperation at the end of the year. Bring in a small treat for each child, such as some candy with a note reading "Thanks for being so sweet."

OLDER CHILDREN

By the time your child enters junior high, many things which were previously big issues may no longer be problems at all.

> *At my son's junior high, for instance, food is not allowed in the classrooms anyway. This simple fact eliminated a whole host of "how to keep the classroom safe" issues. In addition, I was able to obtain permission for Jason to carry his emergency medication in a fanny pack. This eliminated all of the "where should we keep the medicine pack and how many should we have on campus" questions. There is no "playground time," there are far fewer spills in the lunch area, his classmates generally manage to eat their lunch without wearing it, cooking class is optional, etc. In many ways things do get easier at this age.*

Once your child enters the junior high and high school environment, you may need to take steps to ensure that her brought-from-home lunch remains in her possession and untouched by other students until lunchtime. Many schools no longer have lockers, and in some schools the lockers that the students use during physical education classes are not big enough to hold backpacks, books, and lunches (which are simply placed on top of the lockers during class). Make sure that your child's "safe" lunch is either in her possession or locked up until lunch time. Do not make her lunch accessible to "practical jokers" who may tamper with it in some way.

If your child wears her medication to school in a fanny pack, you may need to make arrangements for her to lock this fanny pack up in a secure location (such as a gym locker) during physical education class. Many children find it difficult to run, jump, and fully participate in physical education classes with a fanny pack banging against their body. If your child does remove her fanny pack for this class, you need to make arrangements for her physical education teacher to carry a back-up medicine pack during your child's class time, especially if class is held out on a field, away from the locker room. Of course, you must also have a plan for ensuring that your child remembers to put the fanny pack back on after class is over!

TEASING

Although children can be very compassionate and understanding, your child may eventually encounter teasing about his condition or something relating to his condition (such as his EpiPen® fanny pack or his special peanut-free lunch table).

"TEASING" VS. "QUESTIONING"

Teach your child that there is a difference between "teasing" and "questioning." Other children will naturally be curious about your child's allergies. You can role-play with your child so that she is comfortable giving factual answers to these polite questions. Teasing, on the other hand, is malicious – not polite – and requires a different type of response.

SNAPPY COMEBACK LINES

Children will often stop teasing if they see that your child is not upset. For this reason, you may want to help your child to think of some "snappy comeback lines" to use in these situations.

> *When my son entered a new school for seventh grade, he found himself on the receiving end of some snide remarks about his fanny pack (in which he carries two EpiPens® and some liquid antihistamine). On the first day of school he found this very hurtful. But by day two he was prepared. When the same chil-*

dren taunted "Where'd you get your fanny pack (laugh, laugh, snicker, snicker)" he loudly replied "Why? Would you like one, too?" When others teased "Why are you wearing that stupid fanny pack?" he confidently looked them in the eye and said "I'm starting a new fad." The teasing didn't last for long.

TEASING IS NOT ACCEPTABLE

Of course, teasing at school is not acceptable and can become a form of harassment. If your child is the object of teasing, the teacher and/or school administration should be notified. If your child is not able to stop the teasing through her (non-violent!) actions, it is the school's responsibility to put a stop to this unacceptable behavior.

In my case, in addition to giving my son some ideas for ways to handle the rude remarks, I also trooped straight to the school office to alert the vice principal that there may be a problem. He assured me that if the teasing continued and became a problem, the school would meet with the teasing students to address the issue. As it turns out, the boy who initially started the teasing on the first day of school also has food allergies (although not as severe as Jason's). The two of them became friends and wound up eating lunch together every day for months!

CARPOOLS

If you would like to participate in a carpool ("school run") for your child, there are a few things which you need to keep in mind:

✦ All of the other drivers in the carpool need to be fully trained in how to recognize and treat an allergic reaction.

✦ Your child's medicine pack needs to be in the car with your child.

✦ Many families do a great deal of eating in their cars, resulting in surfaces that are covered in food residue. If this is a concern, arrange to have your child sit on a clean beach towel while in other people's cars, and instruct your child to try not to touch anything.

COLLEGE

When choosing the right college for your child, food allergies are one of the important factors which you need to consider. There are a number of issues that you will need to address, including:

✦ Will there be any safe food for your child to eat at the dining hall?

✦ Where is the nearest hospital?

✦ Is there an on-campus clinic – and, if so, are they equipped to handle an anaphylactic reaction?

———— ✦ ————

FAAN has published an excellent booklet titled "A College Guide for the Student with Food Allergies: It's Not All Pizza and Ice Cream." This publication features a "college time line" guide to assessing colleges (from the allergy perspective) which begins in the summer between your child's last two years of High School and concludes with the first month of college; advice for dealing with social situations; and some insights from food allergic adults. You can order the booklet at www.foodallergy.org.

NOTES

CHAPTER 13

EXTRACURRICULAR ACTIVITIES

Although it will probably require a relatively high level of involvement on your part, your child can participate in sports teams and scouts, take music lessons, and participate in other normal childhood activities. Many food-allergic children even safely go to sleepover camps! This chapter will discuss some of the issues that need to be addressed to make these things happen for your child.

TEACH THE ADULTS IN CHARGE ABOUT YOUR CHILD'S FOOD ALLERGIES

Scout leaders, sports coaches, music teachers, and other adults in charge of your child's extracurricular activities all need to be aware of your child's food allergies. Teach these people what precautions are necessary to keep your child safe, and what to do if your child has an allergic reaction while in their care (see Chapter 2 regarding teaching others about your child's food allergies).

YOU MAY NEED TO BE PRESENT

Be aware that teachers and leaders of extracurricular activities – many of whom are volunteers – may not be willing to take responsibility for your child's safety. They may feel that they are not capable of properly supervising your child in addition to the other children in the group, or they may simply be unwilling to do so. There is no legal requirement that adults in charge of extracurricular activities take this responsibility. It may be best if you plan to be present while your child participates in these activities.

As long as you're going to be present, make yourself useful. Volunteer to assist in some way. Depending on the activity, your child may feel awkward if you're the only parent just standing around at the back of the room – but having one's parent be the official "assistant" may be a source of pride.

CHILDREN'S SPORTS TEAMS

ENROLLMENT FORMS

When you sign your child up for participation on a sports team, be sure to highlight (such as with a yellow highlighting pen) the place on the enrollment form where you have described his food allergies.

YOUR CHILD'S MEDICALERT® BRACELET

As a safety rule, most children's sports programs do not permit the participants to wear jewelry...and many consider your child's MedicAlert® bracelet to be "jewelry." If you remove the bracelet for games, however, you run the risk of losing it, forgetting to put it back on, or not having it in place during an actual medical emergency during or after the game. It also sets a bad precedent, as your child should be taught to wear the bracelet at all times. As a compromise, the sports league may permit you to cover the bracelet with a wrist-sized elasticized sweat band during games. Alternatively, you can purchase a "sports band"-style bracelet directly from the MedicAlert® organization.

ATTEND THE PRACTICES AND GAMES

Unless there is another adult present who has been trained in recognizing and treating an allergic reaction – and has agreed to take on the responsibility of watching your child – you need to stay for all of your child's team practices and team games. Even if your child does not eat anything, you need to assess the risk that he will come in contact with and react to the food residue that is on the other players' hands, especially as many sports involve a high degree of physical contact.

———❧———

Even if you have made the commitment to be there for every one of your child's team practices and team games, it is still a good idea to teach the coach and assistant coach how to recognize and treat an allergic reaction. In case you should be in the restroom or on the other side of the field chasing your toddler when a reaction happens, someone else should know what to do in an emergency.

TALK TO THE OTHER PARENTS

At the first parents' meeting of your child's sports team, explain your child's situation to the other parents. Ask the other parents to please have their children wash their hands prior to coming to team practices and games. In most sports teams the parents take turns bringing snacks for the children. Volunteer to be the "snack coordinator."

TEAM SNACKS

In most team sports, the parents take turns bringing in snacks for all of the children on the team. If this is the case, there are three main options for how to handle snacks, and each has its drawbacks. See page 130 (in the "Preschool" chapter) for a discussion of each option.

————✦————

If you choose to distribute a list of safe snacks to the other parents, keep in mind that you do not need to limit the list to items that your child actually likes. You can lengthen the list by including all child-friendly snack foods that are safe.

> *Diane's food-allergic son successfully participates in many sports teams. She speaks to the coach before the season begins, makes an announcement at the first parents' meeting, and distributes a list of safe snacks. Diane always tells the other parents that if their child has a favorite snack that is not on the approved list, she would be happy to check the ingredients to see if it can be added. The feedback Diane receives is that her list actually makes snack buying easier for other parents. They don't have to think about what to purchase. They just pick something from the list.*

————✦————

> *Laura ends her written letter about safe snacks which she sends to the parents of her son's teammates by saying "Thank you so much for your kindness in this regard. And thanks for letting us play with such a great group of kids!"*

GIRL SCOUTS AND BOY SCOUTS

FOOD AT MEETINGS

If your child's scout troop serves snacks at meetings, the same issues apply as with snacks for sports teams. See above.

————✦————

Many popular children's art and science projects involve food items. Work with your child's scout leader to ensure that no allergenic foods are used in planned activities.

CAMPOUTS

A highlight of many scouting programs is weekend camping. In order to make this a safe activity for your child, you and the scout leader need to address the following issues:

❑ What food will be served on the campout? Is it possible to only serve food to all of the children that is safe for your child?

❑ If allergenic food will be served on the campout, how can you ensure that it won't "contaminate" your child's food, all of the children will wash their hands immediately after eating, and all allergenic food residue will be properly cleaned up from the campsite?

❑ If you are going to be sending separate food for your child, how will it be kept safe, fresh, and separate from everyone else's food?

❑ In case your child does have an allergic reaction, how quickly can he be transported to the nearest hospital emergency room? If the troop will be camping in a remote area, it is probably not a safe situation for your child.

❑ Will your child be carrying his emergency medication in a fanny pack?

❑ Who will carry an extra medicine pack?

❑ Who will be responsible for keeping an eye on your child, and being immediately available to treat him in case he does have a reaction?

❑ Should the entire troop – adults and children – be given some emergency training? Perhaps this can be done in the context of "first aid training."

GIRL SCOUT FOOD ALLERGY PATCH PROGRAM

If your child is an American Girl Scout, you may want to look into the "Be a PAL" food allergy patch program. Details about how the members of your child's troop can earn this patch can be downloaded from FAAN's website, www.foodallergy.org, or from www.gscnc.org (the website of the Girl Scout Council of the Nation's Capital).

CAMPS IN GENERAL

To a large degree, many of the issues that must be addressed to create a safe school environment are also pertinent for your child's camp experience. What steps will the camp take to prevent an allergic reaction? Who will be trained to treat an allergic reaction, and who will train these people? Where will the medication be kept? Will there be any food-related crafts or projects which might not be safe for your child? And so forth. Therefore, I recommend you read Chapter 12 before you read this section. In addition, there are some issues which are more specific to the camp environment, such as concerns about food preparation and (if the camp is in a rural or remote area) concerns about the availability of emergency medical treatment.

DAY CAMPS

For your child's first camp experience, it is probably best if you choose a "day camp" (a camp which only operates during daytime hours, from which your child comes home every afternoon or evening). Preparing a day camp to care for your child is really strikingly similar to preparing a school to care for your child.

SEND YOUR CHILD'S FOOD TO DAY CAMP

You will greatly decrease your child's chance of an allergic reaction if you arrange to send all of your child's food from home. However, even if your child is not going to be eating any of the food supplied by the day camp, it is helpful for the staff to know which of the camp-provided snacks and meals are allergenic for your child and which are not. If they are serving an allergenic food to the rest of the group, they will know to be extra careful with the clean-up. Make arrangements to go into the day camp's kitchen once or twice a week (depending on how frequently they purchase food supplies) and apply the same "red and green dot" food marking system which you may be using in your own home (see page 51).

SLEEPOVER CAMPS AND OVERNIGHT SCHOOL TRIPS

At some point in time your child may become interested in "sleepover" camp, or overnight trips may become part of the curriculum at your child's school. Once again, just like everything else, sending your child to sleepover camp is do-able but requires advance preparation.

———————✒————————

If your child is participating in an overnight trip with her school, meet with the school administrators prior to the trip to find out who will be on the trip, who will be eating with the students, whether there is adult supervision of the sleeping arrangements, and who will be responsible for your child's safety (from the food allergy perspective).

MAKING SLEEPOVER CAMP SAFE FOR YOUR CHILD

The Food Allergy and Anaphylaxis Network has addressed the "camp" topic in their newsletter, on their website, and in a booklet[1]. Among other things, FAAN recommends that you:

---

[1] Food Allergy Newsletter Volume Seven, Number Four, April-May 1998, page 3; Food Allergy Newsletter Volume Three, Number Five, June-July 1994, page 3; FAAN website, www.foodallergy.org, "Managing Food Allergies at Camp."

❑ Choose a camp with a low student-to-camp counselor ratio so your child will be assured of immediate attention, if needed.

❑ Visit the camp. Meet with the camp director and the staff members responsible for food preparation. Visit the kitchen and read ingredient labels for all foods that will be served. Discuss cross-contamination issues, dish washing methodology, and all of the things which you would normally discuss with a restaurant manager (see Chapter 9).

❑ Educate the camp staff about how to prevent, recognize and treat a reaction. Be sure to include the camp director, cook, dining hall/cafeteria workers, cabin director, counselors, camp nurses, swimming pool life guards, transportation drivers, specialty area workers, and anyone else who may offer food or plan activities or events.

❑ Call the emergency response team that would dispatch the ambulance for camp. Find out if the ambulance carries epinephrine at all times or if it must be requested. What is the expected wait time for the ambulance?

❑ Speak with the Emergency Room department of the local hospital and fax or mail all the information necessary to register your child in an emergency. Include your child's camp dates.

❑ Provide copies of your written emergency plan (see Appendix B) to the camp director and camp counselors.

❑ Educate and review with your child the self-management of his food allergy. Your child should know safe and unsafe foods, strategies for avoiding exposure to unsafe foods, symptoms of allergic reactions, how and when to tell an adult about a possible allergic reaction, and how to use his EpiPen®. Your child should know to never trade food with other campers, to never eat anything with unknown ingredients or food preparation methods, and to never go off alone if symptoms are beginning.

———— ❧ ————

For more FAAN camp resources, including both downloadable and for-purchase materials, visit FAAN's website at www.foodallergy.org. I recommend their "Preparing for Camp and Overnight School Trips With Food Allergies" booklet.

SEND MORE THAN ONE MEDICINE PACK

Talk to the camp staff to determine how many medicine packs you should send with your child, and where these will be kept. Your child should wear a fanny pack with one set of emergency medication. You may want to have additional medicine packs in the camp cafeteria and with your child's camp counselor.

CONSIDER SENDING FOOD FROM HOME

If your child has severe, multiple food allergies, you may find it safest to make arrangements to send most or all of your child's food from home to the sleepover camp. In this case, you would prepare your child's meals in advance, freeze this food, and send it with your child to camp. The camp personnel would then be responsible for safely storing, thawing and heating this food for your child.

———————

However, don't rule out the possibility of the camp chef cooking for your child until you talk to him or her.

My son Jason had a fabulous experience at a 5-day science camp with his sixth grade class. I called the chef, Joe, two months before the trip, expecting to make arrangements to send all of Jason's food from home. (Visiting the camp in person was not an option due to the camp's location.) To my surprise, Joe insisted that the camp could handle preparing safe meals for Jason. Joe assured me that he would personally cook Jason's food, and that he was accustomed to handling many special dietary needs.

We discussed ingredients and cross-contamination. Joe promised that peanut butter would not be served to anyone during Jason's stay. Joe assured me that the entire staff had already received EpiPen® training, due to the high number of peanut-allergic campers that had come before Jason, and that many of the counselors were trained medics. I found out that the camp included one food-related activity, and Joe assured me that he would purchase the brand and variety of this food that Jason was not allergic to. I also learned that in an emergency Jason could be airlifted to a major hospital and be there within 15 minutes. The end result: Jason went to science camp and had the time of his life, while I stayed home and spent the week worrying for nothing!

NOTES

CHAPTER 14

MISCELLANEOUS MEDICAL ISSUES

DON'T DO ALLERGY TESTING AT HOME

Allergy testing should only be done under proper medical supervision. Do NOT ever intentionally feed your child an allergen to see if he has outgrown the allergy. Do not do a "home challenge."

> *At the time that I was finishing this manuscript, I took my 13-year-old son to the allergist's office for a controlled food challenge. For this test, the nurse mixes measured amounts of egg protein powder with applesauce, and feeds it to the child; if there is no reaction after thirty minutes the test is repeated with twice as much protein powder. This continues every half hour until a specific amount of protein has been consumed. The result of this test: three minutes after consuming the equivalent of $1/72^{nd}$ of an egg, Jason had an anaphylactic reaction. His throat began to close up, his tongue itched, and he felt as though the inside of his ear was closing up. Let me repeat this. I saw for myself that $1/72^{nd}$ of an egg (what is this – a "half a crumb"?) can cause an anaphylactic reaction in a matter of minutes. Do not purposely feed allergens to your child at home!*

DENTISTS

Be sure that your child's dentist is aware of your child's food allergies. Call the dentist's office a few weeks in advance of your child's appointment to check on the ingredients of all of the products that the dentist would be putting in your child's mouth. If necessary, call the product manufacturers to verify the safety of these items. Repeat this procedure prior to each of your child's dental appointments.

FLU SHOTS

As of this writing, influenza vaccines are grown on egg embryos, and therefore may contain a small amount of egg protein. The standard disclaimer that you must sign prior to receiving these shots states that influenza vaccines are not safe for those with egg allergy. Talk to your child's doctor to determine the safety and appropriateness of the flu shot for your child.

MEDICATIONS

Be sure to check the ingredients (especially the "inactive ingredients") of both prescription and over-the-counter medications prior to giving them to your child. To find the ingredient statements of prescription medications ask your pharmacist for a copy of the medication's manufacturer's package insert. Many medications contain lactose as a sweetener. Some asthma medications contain soy-based propellants. Don't assume that medications are safe for your child – or that the doctor who wrote the prescription was aware of all of the medication's ingredients.

GENERAL ANESTHETICS

Some general anesthetics, including those popular in pediatrics, contain food ingredients. If your child is having a procedure which requires general anesthetic, you must specifically discuss your child's allergies with the anesthesiologist prior to the day on which the procedure is scheduled. Do not assume that that the anesthesiologist is aware of the ingredients of the anesthesia or your child's allergies. Insist that he or she double-checks the medication's safety for your child.

HOSPITALIZATION

What if your food-allergic child needs to be hospitalized (perhaps for a condition or situation totally unrelated to her allergies)? I know that this is something that I have worried about, although thankfully my son has never been hospitalized. What steps can you take to prevent your child from having an allergic reaction while at the hospital? This is a topic that the Food Allergy & Anaphylaxis Network has addressed in past issues of the Food Allergy Newsletter[1]. These articles explain:

✦ With rare exceptions, hospital food is prepared in huge kitchens in massive quantities by people who may not understand food allergy.

---

[1] Food Allergy Newsletter, Volume Ten, Number Six, August-September 2001, page 5; and Food Allergy Newsletter, Volume Three, Number One, October-November 1993, page 3.

✦ You should note the food allergy on your child's medical record, speak directly with the hospital dietician to discuss special dietary needs, and post a sign on your child's door that alerts the staff not to serve a tray until it has been checked by a specified, designated person – preferably you.

✦ Even when a child's hospital chart indicates the presence of a food allergy, parents must always remain vigilant about possible exposure to "unsafe" foods.

✦ Check the trays before they are served to your child. Be suspicious of foods that are prepared with multiple ingredients. If you are unable to speak with a member of the dietary staff regarding a questionable item, avoid that food.

✦ If your child is on a liquid diet, ask what the liquid is made of.

✦ Upon admission, review your child's emergency plan with the admitting nurse. In the event your child does have a reaction, this ensures that emergency medications will be readily available in the correct dosages.

✦ Let everyone on the unit (including staffers on various shifts) know about your child's food allergy.

✦ If you do not feel confident that the hospital can provide safe, "uncontaminated" food for your child, another option is for you to bring safe, non-perishable food items to the hospital and have these available for your child as snacks and meal substitutions.

✦ Be aware of potential exposures beyond meal trays. There may be food debris on bedside tables and in common areas (such as the playroom); coffee cups containing milk are left everywhere; candies at the nurse's station; visitors who come bearing gifts of food; and trash cans contain leftover food items and food wrappers.

DOCTORS – RED FLAGS

Not all Board Certified Allergists have experience in diagnosing and caring for children who have severe, potentially anaphylactic food allergies. Most are quite knowledgeable about asthma and environmental allergies, but not all are up-to-date in their knowledge of food allergies. If your child's physician does any of the following, you may want to find a different allergist:

✦ States that positive food allergy skin prick tests are 100% accurate (as of this writing, they are not – skin prick tests are known to result in a fairly large percentage of false positive results for food allergy testing).

✦ On the basis of skin prick tests alone, advises you to completely remove food from your child's diet that your child has successfully and regularly been eating without incident.

✦ Does not prescribe epinephrine (such as an EpiPen®) for a child who has had a previous anaphylactic reaction.

✦ Prescribes an EpiPen®, but does not teach you how and when to use it.

"MIRACLE CURES"

Be wary of non-traditional medical practitioners who claim that they can "cure" your child's food allergies. As of this writing, there is no "cure" for food allergies – although progress is being made on various treatments which would greatly lessen an allergic reaction if a small amount of allergen was accidentally eaten.

Jackie in Australia considered (and decided against) taking her son to a woman who claimed she had a strong track record of curing peanut allergy in the U.S. Part of her treatment involves placing a "safe" amount of allergen on the child's skin. The woman's advertising materials did not mention the fact that, depending on the severity of the child's allergies, even touching a small amount of allergen can cause a reaction.

———— ✐ ————

I myself went to a Chinese doctor to try acupuncture as a cure for my severe multiple environmental allergies. He started with some unusual diagnostic tests that involved my holding a glass vial of allergens in one hand while resisting physical pressure with my other arm. After six weeks of acupuncture treatments (which also involved my avoiding certain allergens for specified lengths of time and my taking herbal pills) he repeated the tests and announced that I was completely cured. This was a surprise to me, as my symptoms and my reactions remained unchanged.

CHAPTER 15

FOOD ALLERGY SUPPORT GROUPS

If at all possible, join or start a local support group for parents of children with severe food allergies. Caring for a child with life-threatening food allergies is very difficult. A support group can provide emotional support from other parents who are facing similar challenges, and provides a forum for sharing of resources, ideas and experiences. It is truly wonderful to be able to meet with other parents who really "get it."

 INTERNATIONAL PERSPECTIVE

COUNTRY	COMMENTS
Canada	Anaphylaxis Canada can refer you to an established support group within your community, or provide you with a resource kit to help you set up your own. Visit www.anaphylaxis.ca for details.
United Kingdom	The Anaphylaxis Campaign has a network of (volunteer) regional contacts throughout the U.K., as well as a full-time (paid) national coordinator.

SUPPORT GROUP STRUCTURE

There are many different ways in which a support group can be structured. Some groups, such as mine, are very informal, and focus on discussions of allergy-related issues and questions raised by individual members. Other groups regularly feature guest speakers (such as doctors, nutritionists, psychologists, chefs and school nurses) at their meetings. Many groups plan topics for each meeting. Your group may choose to devote its energies to outreach efforts such as fund raising or legislative advocacy. The possibilities are endless.

SUPPORT GROUP SOCIAL EVENTS

PARTIES

Imagine taking your child to the buffet table at a party and telling him that all of the food is "safe"... he can eat whatever he wants. And then imagine letting your child wander off on his own at that same party, with you only supervising him to the same degree that most parents keep an eye on their children at a party... no trailing along right next to him, no worrying about what his playmates are eating or what he's touching. With the help of your support group, you can make this fantasy come true.

————— ❧ —————

Your support group can create family parties at which every child in attendance can eat every food item served. Our support group does this twice a year, and it's wonderful. In order to ensure that the party menu takes all of the party attendees' needs into account, we have a policy requiring those who wish to attend the party to either attend the party-planning meeting or RSVP prior to this meeting. At the meeting we determine the general menu "ground rules" based on the common allergies that we're dealing with (such as no dairy, egg, nut, wheat, or citrus fruits). We then brainstorm food ideas, with each party attendee having veto power over any food idea that is put forth.

————— ❧ —————

Of course, each of us is "extra careful" to check ingredients and avoid cross-contamination when preparing food for these parties.

————— ❧ —————

Our support group has an annual Halloween Party featuring "safe" food, a costume parade, crafts and activities. One of these activities is trick-or-treating for non-food "treats" (such as pencils, small plastic toys, etc.). When our group was small enough to hold the party in someone's home, this activity was really quite special. Each of the mothers would stand inside one of the bedrooms, bathrooms, or closets of the house with her basket of treats. The fathers would then bring the children around the house in small groups. The kids would get to knock on the doors and "trick or treat" for their prizes (which they placed in bags that they had decorated earlier in the party at the crafts table).

> *One year we had to accommodate so many different allergies at our support group's annual Halloween Party that we ended up serving carrots three different ways just to make it look like more of a spread! We had eliminated nuts, animal products of all kinds (including dairy, egg, meat, poultry, fish, and gela-*

tin), all grains except rice, and most fruits and vegetables. We served shredded carrots, carrots cut into little flower shapes, and baby carrots dipped in guacamole. We rounded out the menu with apple slices sprinkled with cinnamon sugar, rice crackers with jam, a cooked rice dish, a big bowl of black olives, and bananas. And it was a fabulous party!

For older children, a "food allergy quiz game" is also a popular party activity.

Support group family social events are a great opportunity for your child to meet other children with food allergies. Children like to see that they are not alone, that there is a whole group of children in their area who also must be careful about what they eat, carry medication, and wear MedicAlert® bracelets!

BAKED GOODS EXCHANGES

Another popular event that our group holds is our annual Baked Goods Exchange. This meeting, for parents only, is held at someone's home. Each member bakes up a large batch of something that is safe for their child, and that meets our ground rules of being nut-, dairy-, and egg-free (as the majority of our members' children have these allergies). The member comes to the meeting with a tray of individually wrapped baked goods, a "tasting tray" of the item made, copies of the recipe, and information about all of the ingredients. At the meeting each attendee distributes her recipe, describes in detail exactly what is in the dish (i.e., the ingredients of the margarine, the sprinkles, etc.), and passes the tasting tray. We all have a great time sampling each item, and then we each fill a bakery box with a few of each treat that is safe for our children. Because our children cannot eat things from bakeries, enjoy dessert buffets, and so forth, this is their one opportunity to enjoy a whole assortment of cookies and cakes.

OTHER ACTIVITY IDEAS

Ideas for family activities include parties and picnics, children's play groups, bowling or miniature golf outings, family camping trips, fund raising events, and babysitting co-ops. Be sure to include siblings, too.

COMPARE PANTRY CONTENTS

A great way to get new ideas for what to feed your child is to get together with one of your support group friends whose child has the same allergies as your child, to see what is in her pantry and what is in her refrigerator. You may be surprised by the variety of locally-available "safe" products that she has found of which you were not aware.

CHILDREN'S GROUP THERAPY SESSIONS

Many children have difficulty dealing with the emotional side of coping with food allergies. It's not easy being different, and it's not easy living with the stress of always having to be so careful about seemingly everything. Your support group may want to make arrangements with a competent local mental health professional for group therapy sessions for your children.

STARTING AND RUNNING A SUPPORT GROUP

If there is no existing support group in your area for parents of children with severe food allergies, I highly recommend that you take it upon yourself to start one. Although this may sound like a daunting task, it is really quite do-able. The benefits of having and belonging to a support group include emotional support from others who are in similar circumstances; a forum in which to share resources, ideas and experiences; and new friendships for both you and your children. This section will give you some advice on how to go about getting your new group started.

ARRANGE FOR A MEETING ROOM

Make arrangements for a room in which to hold your group's meetings. A local community center room or meeting room in a local restaurant is ideal. Many hospitals have meeting rooms that are available as well. It is best to avoid meeting in members' homes, so that the meeting is not affected by that person's availability.

You will probably want to plan to hold your meetings without the children, so that the members will be able to speak freely. Your children should not hear you complain about how difficult it is to care for them, and they may be frightened by some of the subjects that are discussed (such as accounts of other children's anaphylactic episodes).

ADVERTISE YOUR NEW GROUP

Create a simple flyer with a brief description of your group. See Appendix I for a sample flyer.

————❧————

Advertise your group's formation by talking to local allergists, pediatricians, school nurses, mothers groups, daycare centers, and organizers of children's play groups. Ask them to help you distribute your flyer. Contact the local chapter of La Leche League (a group that offers support for breast feeding mothers). Obtain permission to post your flyer on the bulletin boards of local hospitals and churches. Spread the news through word of mouth; network with friends, neighbors, acquaintances. There are bound to be others in your area who would be interested in joining. Your job is to find them!

————❧————

Even if only one guest shows up for your first meeting, don't despair. A support group of two is much better than no support group at all. Once you get started your group is bound to grow.

YOUR GROUP'S FIRST MEETING

At your first meeting you should:

❑ Have each person fill out a name tag and sign a sign-in sheet upon arrival.

❑ Have each person introduce herself and tell about her child's allergies.

❑ Discuss the purpose and goals of the group.

❑ Determine who will be the group's leader; this person will lead meetings and be the group's contact person.

❑ Divide responsibilities and encourage active involvement. People will be more supportive of an organization which they help create. Have others suggest topics and speakers, take responsibility for member communications, do research, offer sample recipes or products, and bring up issues.

❑ Discuss how the members want to structure the meetings... free form vs. formal vs. something in between.

❑ Obtain contact information (including name, address, phone number, e-mail address, and children's names, ages and allergies) for each person present.

❑ Set up a method for communicating with each other, such as distribution of the group's roster and creation of an e-mail distribution list.

STRUCTURE OF MY SUPPORT GROUP

Here is how my support group is structured:

✦ We meet monthly, in the meeting room of a local restaurant. One member of our group is responsible for reserving this room.

✦ Membership in our group is completely free.

✦ About a week before the meeting we send out an e-mail reminder about the meeting date. One member of our group is responsible for maintaining the e-mail distribution list and sending out these reminders.

✦ At the meeting, a dry erase board is placed at the front of the room. This agenda board is divided into two sections: "Announcements" and "Issues." "Announcements" are items that do not require discussion, and that will take about 2 minutes or less. Examples of announcements include new products, recipes, news about good test results, etc. "Issues" are everything else – anything which will require discussion or for which the member is hoping to gain advice. Examples of "issues" include problems at school, travel issues, coping issues, difficulties with parties and social events, problems with friends and relatives, upsetting new diagnoses, etc.

✦ As members arrive at the meeting, those who would like to be on the agenda and share something with the group write their names on the board in the appropriate sections.

✦ The meeting time is then allocated based on how many items are on the agenda board. This system ensures that everyone who has something to share or discuss gets a chance to do so.

✦ As the group leader it is my job to keep the discussion on track and on subject. It is very easy for a group of very emotional women to digress into side issues, but when this happens we run the risk of not having enough time to devote to the items that are on the agenda. I believe that if a member comes to a meeting with a problem, the group needs to devote the necessary time to helping her.

✦ Our meetings occasionally feature guest speakers, but we have found that what our members want and need most is a forum for discussing the issues that arise in coping with our children's severe food allergies.

APPENDICES

APPENDIX A:
RESOURCES

In addition to the organizations listed here, please visit my website, www.FoodAllergyBooks.com, for links to various food allergy-related products (such as books, clothing, EpiPen® carrying devices, and food products) and information.

ORGANIZATIONS IN THE UNITED STATES

ALLERGY AND ASTHMA NETWORK/MOTHERS OF ASTHMATICS, INC. (AANMA)
2751 Prosperity Ave., Suite 150
Fairfax, VA 22031
703-573-7794
800-878-4403
www.aanma.org

AMERICAN ACADEMY OF ALLERGY, ASTHMA AND IMMUNOLOGY (AAAAI)
611 East Wells Street
Milwaukee, WI 53202
414-272-6071
Patient information and physician referral line: 800-822-2762
www.aaaai.org

ASTHMA AND ALLERGY FOUNDATION OF AMERICA
1233 - 20th Street, NW, Suite 402
Washington, DC 20036
800-727-8462
202-466-7643
www.aafa.org

FOOD ALLERGY & ANAPHYLAXIS NETWORK (FAAN)
11781 Lee Jackson Hwy.,
Suite 160
Fairfax, VA 22033-3309
800-929-4040
www.foodallergy.org

FOOD ALLERGY INITIATIVE
625 Madison Avenue, 11th Floor
New York, NY 10022
212.527.5835
www.foodallergyinitiative.org

INTERNATIONAL ASSO-CIATION FOR MEDICAL ASSISTANCE TO TRAVELERS (IAMAT)
417 Center Street
Lewiston, NY 14092
In United States: 716-754-4883
In Canada: 519-836-0102 or
416-652-0137
www.iamat.org

**MEDICALERT
FOUNDATION
INTERNATIONAL**
2323 Colorado Avenue
Turlock, CA 95382
888-633-4298
www.medicalert.org

PEANUTALLERGY.COM
15 Leavitt St.
Long Island ME 04050
207-766-5292
www.peanutallergy.com

ORGANIZATIONS OUTSIDE OF THE UNITED STATES

**MEDICALERT
FOUNDATION
INTERNATIONAL**
Visit website for contact information in various countries
www.medicalert.org

AUSTRALIA
Anaphylaxis Australia Inc.
21 Robinson Close
Hornsby Heights, NSW 2077
1300 728 000
www.allergyfacts.org.au

**Australasian Society of Clinical
Immunology and Allergy Inc.
(ASCIA)**
P.O. Box 450
Balgowah, NSW 2093
0425 216 402
www.allergy.org.au

CANADA
Anaphylaxis Canada
416 Moore Avenue, Suite 306
Toronto, Ontario M4G 1C9
Canada
416-785-5666
www.anaphylaxis.ca

**Allergy/Asthma Information
Association**
Box 100
Toronto, Ontario M9W 5K9
Canada
416-679-9521
800-611-7011
www.aaia.ca

NEW ZEALAND
Allergy New Zealand
1224a Dominion Road, Mt. Roskill
P.O. Box 56-117
Auckland, 1135
0800 34 0800
09 303 2024
www.allergy.org.nz

UNITED KINGDOM
Anaphylaxis Campaign
P.O. Box 275
Farnborough, Hampshire GU146SX
01252 542029
www.anaphylaxis.org.uk

APPENDIX B:
FOOD ALLERGY ACTION PLAN

The following "Food Allergy Action Plan" form can be downloaded for free from the FAAN website, www.foodallergy.org. English and Spanish versions are available.

Food Allergy Action Plan

ALLERGY TO:_____

Student's
Name:_____D.O.B:_____Teacher:_____

Place
Child's
Picture
Here

Asthmatic Yes* ☐ No ☐   *High risk for severe reaction

◆ **SIGNS OF AN ALLERGIC REACTION** ◆

Systems: **Symptoms:**

•**MOUTH**   itching & swelling of the lips, tongue, or mouth
•**THROAT***   itching and/or a sense of tightness in the throat, hoarseness, and hacking cough
•**SKIN**   hives, itchy rash, and/or swelling about the face or extremities
•**GUT**   nausea, abdominal cramps, vomiting, and/or diarrhea
•**LUNG***   shortness of breath, repetitive coughing, and/or wheezing
•**HEART***   "thready" pulse, "passing-out"

The severity of symptoms can quickly change. *All above symptoms can potentially progress to a life-threatening situation.

◆ **ACTION FOR MINOR REACTION** ◆

1. If **only symptom(s) are:**_____, give_____
                                                                    medication/dose/route
_____

Then call:

2. Mother_____, Father _____, or emergency contacts.
3. Dr. _____ at _____

If condition does not improve within 10 minutes, follow steps for Major Reaction below.

◆ **ACTION FOR MAJOR REACTION** ◆

1. **If ingestion is suspected and/or symptom(s) are:**_____,

give_____IMMEDIATELY!
                        medication/dose/route

Then call:

2. Rescue Squad (ask for advanced life support)
3. Mother_____, Father _____, or emergency contacts.
4. Dr. _____ at _____

DO NOT HESITATE TO CALL RESCUE SQUAD!

Parent's Signature_____Date_____ Doctor's Signature_____ Date_____

Reprinted with permission from the Food Allergy and Anaphylaxis Network.

FOOD ALLERGY ACTION PLAN, CONT'D

EMERGENCY CONTACTS	TRAINED STAFF MEMBERS
1. _____	1. _____ Room _____
Relation: _____ Phone: _____	2. _____ Room _____
2. _____	
Relation: _____ Phone: _____	3. _____ Room _____
3. _____	
Relation: _____ Phone: _____	

EPIPEN® AND EPIPEN® JR. DIRECTIONS

1. Pull off gray activation cap.

2. Hold black tip near outer thigh (always apply to thigh).

3. Swing and jab firmly into outer thigh until Auto-Injector mechanism functions. Hold in place and count to 10. The EpiPen® unit should then be removed and taken with you to the Emergency Room. Massage the injection area for 10 seconds.

For children with multiple food allergies, use one form for each food.

The Food Allergy & Anaphylaxis Network

An "Anaphylaxis Action Plan" is also available for free download from the Australasian Society of Clinical Immunology and Allergy at www.allergy.org.au.

APPENDIX C:
RECOGNIZING ALLERGENS ON INGREDIENT LISTINGS

Unfortunately, at least in the U.S., allergenic ingredients are not always listed in "plain English" on product packaging – although most of the major food manufacturers are currently improving their practices in this area.

The following information, which is reprinted from the Food Allergy and Anaphylaxis Network's "How to Read a Label" Cards[1], will help you to determine whether or not a particular product contains ingredients to which your child is allergic. In addition, depending on the severity of your child's allergies, you may also need to consider the possibility that a product that otherwise appears to be "safe" for your child may have been "contaminated" with allergens during the production process. Please see pages 38-42 for a discussion of product cross-contamination.

How to Read a Label for a Milk-Free Diet

Avoid foods that contain milk or any of these ingredients:

+ artificial butter flavor
+ butter, butter fat, butter oil
+ buttermilk
+ casein *(casein hydrolysate)*
+ casseinates *(in all forms)*
+ cheese
+ cream
+ cottage cheese
+ curds
+ custard
+ ghee
+ half & half®
+ lactalbumin, lactalbumin phosphate
+ lactoferrin
+ lactulose
+ milk *(in all forms including condensed, derivative, dry, evaporated, goat's milk and milk from other animals, low-fat, malted, milkfat, non-fat, powder, protein, skimmed, solids, whole)*

+ nougat
+ pudding
+ rennet casein
+ sour cream, sour cream solids
+ sour milk solids
+ whey *(in all forms)*
+ yogurt

May indicate the presence of milk protein:
+ caramel candies
+ chocolate
+ flavorings *(including natural and artificial)*
+ high protein flour
+ lactic acid starter culture
+ lactose
+ luncheon meat, hotdogs, sausages
+ margarine
+ non-dairy products

---

[1] Reprinted with permission from the Food Allergy and Anaphylaxis Network (FAAN), www.foodallergy.org. This information is available for purchase from FAAN in convenient wallet card format.

How to Read a Label for an Egg-Free Diet

Avoid foods that contain eggs or any of these ingredients:

+ albumin *(also spelled as albumen)*
+ egg *(dried, powdered, solids, white, yolk)*
+ eggnog
+ lysozyme
+ mayonnaise
+ meringue *(meringue powder)*
+ surimi

May indicate the presence of egg protein:

+ flavoring *(including natural and artificial)*
+ lecithin
+ macaroni
+ marzipan
+ marshmallows
+ nougat
+ pasta

How to Read a Label for a Peanut-Free Diet

Avoid foods that contain peanuts or any of these ingredients:

+ artificial nuts
+ beer nuts
+ cold pressed, expelled, or extruded peanut oil
+ goobers
+ ground nuts
+ mandelonas
+ mixed nuts
+ monkey nuts
+ nutmeat
+ nut pieces
+ peanut
+ peanut butter
+ peanut flour

May indicate the presence of peanut protein:

+ African, Chinese, Indonesian, Mexican, Thai, and Vietnamese dishes
+ baked goods *(pastries, cookies, etc.)*
+ candy *(including chocolate candy)*
+ chili
+ egg rolls
+ enchilada sauce
+ flavoring *(includes natural and artificial)*
+ marzipan
+ nougat

- Studies show that most allergic individuals can safely eat peanut oil (*not* cold pressed, expelled, or extruded peanut oil).
- Arachis oil is peanut oil.
- Experts advise patients allergic to peanuts to avoid tree nuts as well.
- A study showed that unlike other legumes, there is a strong possibility of cross reaction between peanuts and lupine.
- Sunflower seeds are often produced on equipment shared with peanuts.

How to Read a Label for a Tree Nut-Free Diet

Avoid foods that contain nuts or any of these ingredients:

+ almonds
+ artificial nuts
+ Brazil nuts
+ caponata
+ cashews
+ chestnuts
+ filbert/hazelnuts
+ gianduja *(a nut mixture found in some chocolate)*
+ hickory nuts
+ macadamia nuts
+ mandelonas
+ marzipan/almond paste
+ nan-gai nuts
+ natural nut extract *(such as, almond or walnut extract)*

+ nougat
+ nut butters *(such as cashew butter or almond butter)*
+ nut meal
+ nutmeat
+ nut oil
+ nut paste *(such as almond paste)*
+ nut pieces
+ pecans *(Mashuga Nuts®)*
+ pesto
+ pine nuts *(also referred to as Indian, pinon, pinyon, pignoli, pignolia, and pignon nuts)*
+ pistachios
+ pralines
+ walnuts

• Mortadella may contain pistachios.

• Natural and artificial flavoring may contain tree nuts.

• Experts advise patients allergic to tree nuts to avoid peanuts as well.

• Talk to your doctor if you find other nuts not listed here.

How to Read a Label for a Wheat-Free Diet

Avoid foods that contain wheat or any of these ingredients:

- bran
- bread crumbs
- bulgur
- couscous
- cracker meal
- durum
- farina
- flour *(all purpose, bread, durum, cake, enriched, graham, high gluten, soft wheat, steel ground, stone ground, whole wheat)*
- gluten
- kamut
- matzoh, matzoh meal *(also spelled as matzo)*
- pasta
- scitan

- semolina
- spelt
- vital gluten
- wheat *(bran, germ, gluten, malt, sprouts)*
- wheat grass
- whole wheat berries

May indicate the presence of wheat protein:

- flavoring *(including natural and artificial)*
- hydrolyzed protein
- soy sauce
- starch *(gelatinized starch, modified starch, modified food starch, vegetable starch, wheat starch)*
- surimi

How to Read a Label for a Soy-Free Diet

Avoid foods that contain soy or any of these ingredients:

- edamame
- hydrolyzed soy protein
- miso
- natto
- shoyu sauce
- soy *(soy albumin, soy fiber, soy flour, soy grits, soy milk, soy nuts, soy sprouts)*
- soya
- soybean *(curd, granules)*
- soy sauce

- Tamari
- Tempeh
- textured vegetable protein (TVP)

May indicate the presence of soy protein:

- Asian cuisine
- flavoring *(including natural and artificial)*
- vegetable broth
- vegetable gum
- vegetable starch

• Studies show most individuals allergic to soy may safely eat soy lecithin and soybean oil.

How to Read a Label for a Shellfish-Free Diet

Avoid foods that contain shellfish or any of these ingredients:

+ abalone
+ clams *(cherrystone, littleneck, pismo, quahog)*
+ cockle *(periwinkle, sea urchin)*
+ crab
+ crawfish *(crayfish, ecrevisse)*
+ lobster *(langouste, langoustine, scampo, coral, tomalley)*
+ mollusks
+ mussels
+ octopus
+ oysters
+ prawns
+ scallops

+ shrimp *(crevette)*
+ snails *(escargot)*
+ squid *(calamari)*

May indicate the presence of shellfish protein:

+ bouillabaisse
+ cuttlefish ink
+ fish stock
+ flavoring *(includes natural and artificial)*
+ seafood flavoring *(such as crab or clam extract)*
+ surimi

Keep the following in mind:

• Any food served in a seafood restaurant may be cross-contaminated with fish or shellfish.

• For some individuals, a reaction may occur from cooking odors or from handling fish or shellfish.

 INTERNATIONAL PERSPECTIVE

COUNTRY	COMMENTS
New Zealand	Ingredient Label Cards are also available for purchase from Allergy New Zealand. Go to www.allergy.org.nz to download the resource order form.

APPENDIX D:
SAMPLE LETTERS FROM YOUR DOCTOR
TO CARRY WHEN TRAVELING

INSTRUCTIONS FOR EMERGENCY ROOM PERSONNEL

DATE

To Whom It May Concern:

This is to certify that my patient, NAME, has severe, potentially anaphylactic allergies to LIST OF ALLERGENS GOES HERE.

Patient/patient's parents have been instructed that at the first sign of anaphylaxis he/she should administer epinephrine and NAME OF ANTIHISTAMINE and transport the patient to the Emergency Room.

Emergency Room personnel should: INSTRUCTIONS GO HERE.

After stabilizing, patient must remain under observation at the Emergency Room for a minimum of four (4) hours, as up to 40% of anaphylactic reactions are biphasic.

If you have any questions, I can be reached at TELEPHONE NUMBER.

Sincerely,

_____, MD

MD OFFICE STAMP

AUTHORIZATION FOR CARRYING EPIPENS®
ABOARD COMMERCIAL AIRPLANES

The following letter can be downloaded for free from the FAAN website, www.foodallergy.org.

DATE

To Whom It May Concern:

PATIENT FULL NAME is a AGE/GENDER who suffers from a life-threatening allergy to SPECIFIC ALLERGENS LISTED. This is a severe allergic reaction that makes it medically necessary for HIM/HER to carry an antihistamine and EpiPen®, which is an autoinjector of epinephrine, at all times. EpiPen® autoinjectors are prescribed by a licensed medical professional. PATIENT NAME should have this life-saving medication with HIM/HER at all times, especially during times of travel away from home. In the event of an exposure to even a minute amount of ALLERGEN, a severe allergic reaction may occur. Every minute is critical in using this medication to treat the allergic reaction and to prevent a life-threatening reaction. Use of the EpiPen® can be life saving. Please allow PATIENT NAME to have the EpiPen®(s) with HIM/HER on board the airplane.

{{SUGGESTED TEXT FOR ASTHMATICS}}

PATIENT NAME is also asthmatic and requires the use of an albuterol inhaler in the event of an asthma attack or allergic reaction. Please allow PATIENT NAME to carry HIS/HER albuterol inhaler on board the airplane. Additional information may be obtained from PHYSICIAN NAME at PHONE or FAX.

Respectfully signed,

_____, *M.D.*

M.D. OFFICE STAMP

Reprinted with permission from the Food Allergy and Anaphylaxis Network.

APPENDIX E:
SAMPLE RESTAURANT CARD

In addition to all of the other precautions which you will take when dining at a restaurant (see chapter 9), you may also want to carry a personalized "restaurant card" such as this to give to the chef.

To the Chef:

WARNING! I am severely allergic to _____. In order to avoid a POTENTIALLY FATAL reaction I must avoid all of the following ingredients:

- (List of ingredients goes here)
-
-

Please double-check the ingredients of the food which you are preparing for me, as well as the sub-ingredients of any of these ingredients (for instance, what is in the "bread crumbs"?), to ensure that the food does not contain **anything** to which I am allergic.

My allergies are so severe that I will also have a negative reaction if a food which I am allergic to merely touches my food. Therefore, please also ensure that all utensils and equipment used to prepare my meal, as well as the preparation surfaces, are thoroughly cleaned prior to use.

Thank you very much for your help and cooperation!

APPENDIX F:
SAMPLE AUTHORIZATION FOR CONSENT TO EMERGENCY MEDICAL TREATMENT

AUTHORIZATION TO CONSENT TO TREATMENT OF MINOR

I, the undersigned parent of _____, a minor, do hereby authorize _____ as agent(s) for the undersigned to consent to any X-ray examination, anesthetic, medical or surgical diagnosis or treatment and hospital care which is deemed advisable by, and is to be rendered under the general or special supervision of, any licensed physician or surgeon on the medical staff of any hospital, whether such diagnosis or treatment is rendered at the office of said physician or at said hospital.

It is understood that this authorization is given in advance of any specific diagnosis, treatment or hospital care being required but is given to provide authority and power on the part of the aforesaid agent(s) to give specific consent to any and all such diagnosis, treatment or hospital care which aforementioned physician in the exercise of his/her best judgment may deem advisable.

I hereby authorize any hospital which has provided treatment to the above-named minor to surrender physical custody of such minor to my above-named agent(s) upon the completion of treatment.

These authorizations shall remain effective until _____, unless sooner revoked in writing delivered to said agent(s).

Allergies: _____

Medications child is currently taking: _____

Pediatrician name and phone number: _____

Allergist name and phone number: _____

Date of child's last tetanus toxoid immunization: _____

_____   _____
Parent's Signature   Date

_____   _____
Signature of Witness   Date

APPENDIX G:
SAMPLE LETTER
FROM THE SCHOOL PRINCIPAL

[Date]

Dear Parents,

The new school year will soon be underway, and we are all very excited about the many new things your children will be learning and experiencing. Our school is blessed with an outstanding and diverse community of students, each of whom is unique and special in a variety of ways. This year one [or several] of our students has life-threatening food allergies to peanuts, peanut oil, any product containing peanuts, as well as several other food items.

Children who have life-threatening food allergies look, act, play and learn just like all other children, but they can have a severe – and life-threatening – reaction if they eat, drink, or possibly even come in contact with the food to which they are allergic. This condition is very serious but is not in any way contagious.

In order to provide a safe learning environment, our school will have the following policies:

- All children will wash their hands upon entering the classroom in the morning and after each snack and lunch recess. This will prevent the spread of food residue in the classroom and will also promote good hygiene and help stop the spread of illness.
- No food or drink will be allowed in the classrooms.
- There will be no sharing of food at the lunch tables.
- Class parties and special events will still take place, but will now focus on fun activities rather than on food. If your child is celebrating a birthday, please send non-food items (such as pencils, erasers, or stickers) instead of food treats.

There will also be a special "peanut-free" table in the lunch area. Any student who has brought or purchased a peanut-free lunch is welcome to sit at this table.

Thank you so much for your understanding and support in this very important matter. Please feel free to call the school if you have any questions or concerns.

Sincerely,

[name], Principal

APPENDIX H:
SAMPLE ALLERGY BUTTON ARTWORK

Many crafts stores sell blank 3-inch diameter buttons which you can personalize and then pin onto your toddler or preschooler's clothing whenever you leave the house. Here is some sample artwork which you can photocopy and use, or you can use your creativity to make your own.

Severely Allergic To Peanuts

I Have Food Allergies

PLEASE DO NOT FEED ME

APPENDIX I:
SAMPLE SUPPORT GROUP ANNOUNCEMENT FLYER

FOOD ALLERGY SUPPORT GROUP

NOW FORMING!

Does your child have severe, potentially fatal food allergies?

Would you like to get together with other parents who are facing the same challenges that you are?

Join us.

We will face the challenges together!

For more information, contact:
Name
Phone Number
E-Mail Address

Monthly meetings:
7:00 – 9:00 p.m.
Location Name
Location Address
3rd Monday of each month

APPENDIX J:
CONTACTING FOOD MANUFACTURERS

You may wish to start a notebook in which you keep track of your conversations with food manufacturers. Your notebook should have a separate page for each manufacturer that you contact. Write the company name and telephone number at the top of the page. For each conversation, make a note of the date and time of day on which you called, the name of the person that you spoke to, the products discussed, and what you were told about the safety of these products.

Here is a sample "script" that you can use when contacting a food manufacturer to determine the safety of a particular product. Call the Customer Service telephone number listed on the package.

COMPANY: Good Afternoon, how may I help you?

You: Hi! My name is [name]. I have some questions about the ingredients and possible cross-contamination of [name of specific product].

COMPANY: Yes, ma'am. What is your question?

YOU: My [son/daughter] has very severe, potentially fatal allergies to [list of allergens goes here]. Ingestion of even a minute amount of these things can cause a reaction. Although the ingredient statement of [name of product in question] does not list any [list of allergens goes here] ingredients, I also need to be certain that it is not produced on the same equipment as something else that does contain these things.

[If the ingredient statement includes "natural flavorings" or "artificial flavorings"]: In addition, I need to verify that the "[natural/artificial] flavorings" referred to on the ingredient statement does not contain any of these allergens. Can you address these issues for me or would I need to speak with your supervisor?

COMPANY: (Note: either the customer service representative will be able to answer the question, possibly by reading the company's standard allergy information statements to you, or he/she will refer you to someone else – in which case you need to start all over again. Regardless of what answer is given, question it and repeat it back to the customer service representative to ensure that no mistakes are made.)

YOU: I noticed that the [variety name] variety of this product does contain [allergen]. Are these two varieties produced on different equipment or shared equipment?

COMPANY: (The customer service representative answers your question. If he/she claims that the two varieties are on separate equipment, ask if he/she is quite certain of this fact).

YOU: So you are certain that [product name] is not exposed to any [list of allergens goes here] ingredients at any point in the production process? How about on the packaging equipment?

I need to be quite certain. My son/daughter's well-being is at stake.

OR

Thank you for letting me know that [product name] is produced on the same equipment as [name of other product], which does contain [allergen]. How can I submit an official request to your company that this allergen information be added to your standard product labeling?

APPENDIX K:
SAMPLE "SCRIPT" FOR
CALLING THE RESCUE SQUAD

It is a good idea to keep an emergency "script" by each telephone in your house, for use in case your child has an anaphylactic reaction while at home and someone needs to call for help. It is sometimes difficult during an actual emergency to think clearly regarding what it is you need to say. Here is a sample script. You should modify it as necessary for your circumstances (see pages 19-22).

"This is a medical emergency.

This is (Your Name) at (Your Address) in (Your City).

We have a (X)-year-old child with severe food allergies who is having an anaphylactic reaction.

We have given him his EpiPen® shot.

Please send the paramedics.

Our nearest cross streets are Street Name and Street Name."

APPENDIX L:
RECIPE FOR WHEAT-FREE PLAY DOUGH

1-1/2 cups (187 grams) white rice flour

1 cup (125 grams) salt

2 teaspoons (2.5 grams) Cream of Tartar (this is a white powder which is available in the "spice" section of the supermarket)

1 cup (250 ml) boiling water

1 tablespoon (15 ml) safe cooking oil (such as soy, corn, or canola oil)

15 drops liquid food coloring of your choice

Place rice flour, salt, and Cream of Tartar in a large mixing bowl; mix well. Add water, oil, and food color; stir until cool enough to handle. Remove from bowl and knead for 30 to 45 seconds. Let cool 15 minutes before using.

This will keep for weeks without refrigeration if stored in an airtight container, such as a zipper-type plastic bag.

INDEX

T

CONTACT
THE AUTHOR

Dear Reader,

I sincerely hope that the information presented in this book will help to make it easier for you to manage your child's life-threatening food allergies, and that you will be able to use this book as a handy reference manual for many of the situations that are likely to arise in your life. I know how daunting a task it can be to create and maintain a safe environment for a severely food-allergic child.

I would love to hear from you! Please send me your comments and feedback on *How to Manage Your Child's Life-Threatening Food Allergies.*

I can be reached via e-mail at:

LindaCoss@FoodAllergyBooks.com

Or via snail-mail at:

Linda Coss
Plumtree Press
P.O. Box 1313
Lake Forest, CA   92609-1313

Thank you!

ORDER FORM

Note: Books can also be ordered via credit card from
www.FoodAllergyBooks.com.

Please **photocopy** this form, fill it out, and mail it with payment
(in U.S. dollars only) to:

Plumtree Press
P.O. Box 1313, Dept. B2
Lake Forest, CA   92609-1313

QTY	BOOK TITLE	EACH	TOTAL
	How to Manage Your Child's Life-Threatening Food Allergies	$16.95	
	What's To Eat? The Milk-Free, Egg-Free, Nut-Free Food Allergy Cookbook	$16.95	
	SUBTOTAL		
	Sales Tax: CA residents only add 7.75% tax		
	Shipping and Handling: $3.00/1 book or $4.50/2 books for U.S. 3rd class mail $5.00/1 book or $7.50/2 books for U.S. Priority Mail or Canadian orders $10.00/1 book or $15.00/2 books for shipments to other countries		
	TOTAL:		

Note: Prices and availability subject to change without notice.

Name: _____

Address: _____

_____

E-mail (optional): _____

May 2004